Case Studies in Geriatrics for the House Officer

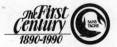

The First Century 1890-1990
SANS TACHE

Case Studies in Geriatrics for the House Officer

Judith C. Ahronheim, M.D.

Clinical Assistant Professor of Medicine
Division of Geriatrics
New York University School of Medicine
New York, New York

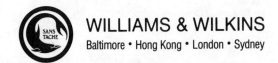

WILLIAMS & WILKINS

Baltimore • Hong Kong • London • Sydney

Editor: Michael G. Fisher
Associate Editor: Marjorie Kidd Keating
Copy Editor: Melissa Andrews
Design: Dan Pfisterer
Illustration Planning: Lorraine Wrzosek
Production: Adele Boyd

Copyright © 1990
Williams & Wilkins
428 East Preston Street
Baltimore, Maryland 21202, USA

Accurate indications, adverse reactions, and dosage schedules for drugs are provided in this book, but it is possible that they may change. The reader is urged to review the package information data of the manufacturers of the medications mentioned.

Printed in the United States of America

Library of Congress Cataloging in Publication Data

Ahronheim, Judith C.
    Case studies in geriatrics for the house officer/Judith C. Ahronheim.
        p. cm. (Case studies for the house officer)
    ISBN 0-683-00064-0
    1. Geriatrics—Case studies.   I. Title.   II. Series.
    [DNLM: 1. Geriatrics—case studies. WT 100 A287c]
RC952.7.A37   1990
618.97'09—dc20
DNLM/DLC
for Library of Congress   89-22696
                                                                                      CIP

        1   2   3   4   5   6   7   8   9   10   89   90   91   92   93

Series Editor's Foreword

The series, Case Studies for the House Officer, has been designed to teach medicine by a case study approach. It is considered a supplement to the parent House Officer Series, which provides information in a problem-oriented format. In CASE STUDIES IN GERIATRICS FOR THE HOUSE OFFICER, Dr. Ahronheim has gathered a series of interesting cases that illustrate the common and unusual problems that confront the house officer who deals with the elderly patient. She has added informative "Pearls" and "Pitfalls" and provocative "Clues." There is a special section on interpreting laboratory values in the geriatric patient. It is hoped that the book will be a useful and enjoyable learning experience for students of the rapidly growing field of geriatrics.

Lawrence P. Levitt, M.D.
Senior Consultant in Neurology
Lehigh Valley Hospital Center
Allentown, Pennsylvania

Clinical Professor of Neurology
Hahnemann University
Clinical Associate Professor
Temple University School of Medicine
Philadelphia, Pennsylvania

To the **Days of the Giants,**

especially

J. Heinz Ahronheim, M.D.
University of Berlin, 1932

Sigmund A. Hirschhorn, M.D.
University of Vienna, 1924

Preface

CASE STUDIES IN GERIATRICS FOR THE HOUSE OFFICER continues the philosophy of the originators of the **HOUSE OFFICER** series. The book will guide physicians and physicians-in-training in recognizing and managing important clinical problems. The case studies approach will propel the reader to think about the total patient, to consider not only the medical but the psychosocial and ethical issues that abound in the management of the elderly, and that are essentially unique to this age group.

Because the field of Geriatrics is one of the newest in the United States, this volume condenses a rapidly growing body of knowledge that faces students, house officers, and practicing physicians alike. But while the body of knowledge and experience expands, eight basic Geriatric Principles endure. The discipline of Geriatric Medicine can only be mastered if the physician is familiar with and understands these important principles.

1. Aging research is handicapped by its own peculiar pitfalls. All studies are hampered by the fact that biologic heterogeneity increases with age, making it practically impossible to find a true control. Healthy people over 85 may represent a biologic elite and their characteristics cannot be extrapolated to all older adults. Cross sectional studies by age group differ in their definition of the age groups under study. Longitudinal studies have their own problems: the findings may be confounded by extrinsic factors that have changed with time.

2. Chronologic and biologic age are imperfectly matched. While some people are "old at 18," many 90-year-olds exhibit behavior (medical and otherwise) that is surprisingly, and sometimes shockingly, youthful. The physician should not view behavior that is simply youthful as "inappropriate," or depression and social crises as "expected at that age." New physical complaints should not be ignored or ascribed simplistically to "old age."
Medical treatment should never be given or withheld on the basis of age alone.

3. <u>Disease more often presents "atypically,"</u> in ways currently not emphasized or even described in most general medical textbooks. This important fact, which will be emphasized repeatedly, is related to the common physiologic and pathologic changes of aging.

4. <u>Older patients often have multiple diseases and functional impairments.</u> Regardless of the age of the patient, the physician should always try to unify multiple symptoms and try to explain them on the basis of one pathologic process. However, in Geriatrics, more often than not, there will be several problems occurring at one time in many organ systems and to different degrees. These problems may be etiologically unrelated, but physiologically intimately interrelated. As such, the physician must not only sharpen "subspecialty" skills, but must become a skillful generalist who can integrate and treat the patient as a unified whole.

5. <u>Silent pathology is often present.</u> Quiescent lesions, such as atherosclerosis, histologic Alzheimer's Disease, or cardiac conduction deficits may remain silent until an additional insult is superimposed or until the organism is stressed. When constructing a patient management strategy, the physician should assume that these lesions are present until proved otherwise.

6. <u>Drugs are potential poisons.</u> On the average, older patients take more drugs, experience more drug-drug interactions, develop more adverse effects, and tend to exhibit a specific spectrum of effects.

7. <u>Geriatrics is a multidisciplinary field.</u> The primary care physician can often not manage the patient without knowledge of and assistance from the fields of social work, psychology, rehabilitation, nursing, nutrition, podiatry, dentistry, and every medical discipline that exists. The geriatrician must occasionally even link up with the pediatrician. The family, if available, is always an integral part of this multidisciplinary team.

8. <u>The primary care physician is the gatekeeper</u> and needs to be aware of and organize all of the people in item 7.

The physician caring for the older patient must master an ever-expanding body of knowledge in this new discipline. Thus, the intent of **CASE STUDIES IN GERIATRICS FOR THE HOUSE OFFICER** is to reach beyond the house officer--to intercept the medical student before non-age-adjusted principles become too firmly imbedded, to remind the house officer to think of the aged patient as potentially different, and to enhance the well-honed skills of the experienced physician. The book should bring to life the principles that are taught in a comprehensive Geriatric textbook. In this way, it should not only serve as a skill-enhancer and a supplemental guide for the Geriatric Certifying Examination, but hopefully will make the learning process enjoyable.

Judith C. Ahronheim, M.D.

Acknowledgments

I would like to thank my NYU faculty colleagues, psychiatrist and psychopharmacologist Istvan Boksay, ophthalmologist Michael Cohen, and neurologist Govindan Gopinathan for their thoughtful reviews of specific sections of this manuscript; physiatrist Valerie Lanyi, for providing input on rehabilitation medicine and photographs for Case 29; radiologist Emil Baltishar for his help in obtaining illustrative material for Cases 11 and 12. I am grateful to the entire staff of the NYU Audiovisual Department for assistance in preparing photographs, to Bob Wilson for his hours of work on many illustrations, and to the photographic group of the Department of Dermatology for their assistance in retrieving photographs for Cases 2, 19, and 22, which are used by permission of the Department of Dermatology, New York University of Medicine. Saul Kamen, Professor of Dental Health at SUNY-Stonybrook, kindly contributed the photograph for Case 11, for which I am happily indebted. Dr. Kamen has been a pioneer in the field of Geriatric Dentistry and was one of my early teachers in Geriatrics. Legal aspects of Cases 8 and 9 were reviewed by Rose Gasner, Staff Attorney, and Elena Cohen, former Staff Attorney of the Society for the Right to Die, an educational and patient advocacy organization with which I have recently become much involved, and whose staff has been of great help in my own understanding of the legal and ethical aspects of Geriatric care. Elena Cohen is currently associated with the New York City law firm, Kalkines, Arky, Zall, & Bernstein, and continues to be an excellent resource on this subject. Finally, I would like to add my name to the multitudes who have acknowledged Professor Hayes Jacobs of the New School for Social Research, New York. He is a great teacher, role model, and gentleman. Thank you, Hayes.

My special thanks go to Gerald Blandford, Professor of Medicine, UMDNJ-Robert Wood Johnson Medical School, computer expert, husband, and geriatrician extraordinaire. Without his uncommon patience and his discovery of the mysteries hidden in my word processing program, this book would not have been at all possible.

The entire manuscript was reviewed by a special group of people, for whom this type of book was originally designed, and I would like to thank them individually. Their studied reviews have been extremely useful and their observations have been incorporated in the final version of this book.

From Internal Medicine:
Joyce Fogel, Geriatrics Fellow
Navneet Kathuria, Resident
New York University
    School of Medicine

From Family Medicine:
Thomas M. Naughton, Geriatrics Fellow
Carol Jackson, Resident
UMDNJ-Robert Wood Johnson
    Medical School

From the Student Body:
Richard Mahr
New York University School of Medicine
Class of 1989

Contents

Part II.

"They didn't know a <u>pupilla</u> from a <u>papilla</u>."

S.A. Hirschhorn

PART I

CASES

Urinary Tract Infection

Case 1. An 84-year-old retired professor was admitted to the coronary care unit of an acute care hospital because of syncope. He had a history of chronic constipation for which he had taken various senna-containing preparations for many years. His most recent bowel regimen also included psyllium hydrophilic mucilloid (Metamucil) twice daily, docusate sodium (Colace) 300 mg daily, and milk of magnesia 30 cc as needed. He had no known history of urinary difficulties.

Physical findings included atrial fibrillation with a ventricular rate of 150, and bibasilar rales. Rectal examination was "deferred." Treatment consisted of digoxin, furosemide, a low salt diet, and Colace 100 mg daily. He was kept on bed rest.

On the second hospital day the patient complained that he was "not being given enough laxatives," and his diet orders were modified to include 10 grams of bran with his breakfast cereal, and two high fiber cookies (5 grams of fiber each) for dessert at lunch and dinner.

By the third hospital day his cardiac status had improved but he began to complain of urinary urgency and inability to void, whereupon it was noted that he had not passed urine for at least 8 hours, although he had been eating and drinking normally. A Foley catheter was inserted and 550 cc of clear urine was passed. The catheter remained in place while cardiac workup proceeded over the next few days.

On the fifth hospital day the patient developed a temperature of 101° F (oral) and urinalysis revealed many bacteria and 8-10 white blood cells per high power field. Urine and blood cultures were sent to the laboratory and ampicillin was begun. The patient began to complain that the catheter was "annoying" him and that it was "probably to blame for the infection in the first place." He demanded that it be removed. The catheter was removed but when the patient was unable to pass urine 8 hours later it was reinserted. He began tugging on the catheter until blood was noted at the urethral meatus, and wrist restraints were ordered by the cardiology fellow. The patient became agitated and a psychiatry consult was called. The patient complained loudly that he was "not senile yet," and would "sue the hospital" unless he could speak to a urologist. The urology resident was called and the problem was promptly resolved.

1

Clue:

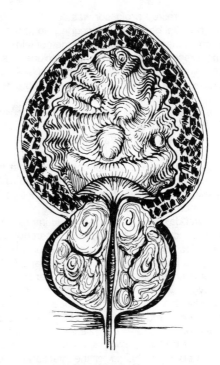

Adapted with permission from Tanagho EA, McAninch JW. Smith's general urology, 12th ed. Norwalk, CT, Appleton and Lange, 1988.

Questions:

1. What factors contributed to the urinary tract infection?

2. What was the most likely cause of the patient's acute urinary retention?

3. What factors led up to this patient's dilemma?

4. What did the urology resident do?

5. What are other causes of acute urinary retention in elderly patients?

Answers:

1. The Foley catheter, acute urinary retention, and statistical likelihood that the patient had underlying benign prostatic hyperplasia probably all contributed to the urinary tract infection. The incidence of catheter-related urinary tract infections increases rapidly with the duration of catheterization at a rate of about 10% per day. In addition, this patient had developed urinary retention prior to catheterization and was already predisposed to infection. Finally, benign prostatic hyperplasia (BPH) is present in at least 80% of men over age 80, and was probably present in this patient, leading to modest chronic retention of urine with stasis and bacteriuria. BPH develops insidiously and patients may not complain of urinary difficulties, many perhaps because they consider urinary hesitancy to be an inevitable problem of old age. The incidence of asymptomatic bacteriuria rises dramatically after midlife in men and is ten times as common in men over 80 than in the 65- to 70-year age group.

2. The patient developed a fecal impaction with a hard mass and accumulation of abundant feces in the rectum, compressing the bladder and resulting in urinary retention. The probability that he had some degree of BPH increased the likelihood that he would develop acute urinary retention.

3. The patient was known to suffer from chronic constipation. His bowel movements occurred to his satisfaction only with a strict bowel regimen. This regimen was not given to him in the hospital, possibly because it was viewed by the staff as an eccentric and excessive use of laxatives. The sudden imposition of bed rest probably reduced his bowel motility further. The diuretic and salt restriction caused relative dehydration and reduced water content of feces, further worsening the patient's bowel function. Although bran has been shown to reduce intestinal transit time in elderly hospitalized patients, bran supplementation can sometimes cause fecal impaction, especially when water content of the diet is not increased, and is relatively contraindicated in bedridden patients. Last but not least, the unfamiliar environment of the hospital with its lack of privacy makes toileting difficult for people of all ages. Defecation into a bed pan is difficult for the hardiest colon to accomplish.

4. The urology resident performed a digital rectal exam and found a rock-hard fecal mass, which he removed, after which the patient expelled soft feces spontaneously. The resident removed the catheter, and, four hours later, the patient urinated on his own. Ideal follow-up treatment should have included saline enemas, bathroom or commode privileges, physical activity as soon as possible, and continuation of the antibiotic to complete a one-week course.

5.   Acute urinary retention, in the absence of spinal cord injury, is usually caused by medications with anticholinergic activity. The detrusor muscle of the bladder contracts in response to cholinergic stimulation, and is inhibited and sometimes paralyzed by anticholinergic agents. Common offenders are the tricyclic antidepressants, antihistamines, gastrointestinal anti-spasmodics (belladonna alkaloids [Donnatal], propantheline [ProBanthine], others), and the antiarrhythmic agent disopyramide (Norpace). Antispasmodics such as oxybutinin (Ditropan) and propantheline are also used to treat urinary incontinence due to spastic (overreactive, hyperreflexic) bladder, and may result in unwanted urinary retention.

Pearls:

1.   Irritant laxatives such as senna directly affect the myenteric plexus. Chronic use of such laxatives can permanently damage the electrical system of the colon. The result is "cathartic bowel," an overdistended colon with loss of haustrations and poor motility. Other irritant laxatives known to cause cathartic bowel include castor oil, cascara, aloe, bisacodyl, and phenolphthalein. Prunes and prune juice contain a phenolphthalein derivative but have not been reported to cause cathartic bowel.

2.   The aged kidney has a blunted response to sodium deficiency so that dietary salt restriction may result in a cumulative sodium deficit. Except in cases of extreme fluid retention, the elderly need not be subjected to salt restriction beyond a 2-gram sodium diet.

Pitfalls:

1.   Bran and high-fiber supplements should not be taken in excess because they may form a bulky mass, thereby increasing constipation and leading to fecal impaction. Whenever the fiber content of a diet is increased, fluid intake should be increased as well, in order to avoid the obstructing mass effect. Bran and high-fiber supplements should not be given at all to bedridden patients who have a high risk of developing an obstructing mass from the fiber.

2.   The rectal examination is important in determining the cause of urinary obstruction but must be interpreted with caution. The size of the prostate gland on digital examination does not necessarily correlate with the degree of obstructive symptoms since the process of adenomatous growth of tissue that characterizes BPH begins in the periurethral area. The prostate may feel relatively normal on digital exam in cases where there may be a high degree of obstruction. Conversely, a patient may have a prostate gland that is large in size but histologically normal and nonobstructing. Prostatic carcinoma tends

to originate in the periphery of the gland and does not usually cause obstructive symptoms early in the course of the disease.

References:

Brandt L. The colon. In: Gastrointestinal disorders of the elderly. New York: Raven Press, 1984:261-367.

Cummings JH. Laxative abuse. Gut 1974;15:758-766.

Epstein M, Hallenberg NK. Age as a determinant of renal sodium conservation in normal men. J Lab Clin Med 1976;87:411-417.

Horton R. Benign prostatic hyperplasia: a disorder of androgen metabolism in the male. J Amer Geriatr Soc 1984;32:380-385.

Kaye D. Urinary tract infections in the elderly. Bull N Y Acad Med 1980;56:209-228.

Pain

Case 2. A 78-year-old healthy woman complains of pain in the left lower back. The pain is burning in nature and has increased in severity over a period of 2 days. On physical examination there is mild local tenderness but normal range of motion and no pain on straight leg raising. Lumbosacral spine films and urinalysis are ordered, and acetaminophen is prescribed.

A week later the patient returns, complaining of a rash and disabling pain in the left side and back. The rash appeared 5 days before. Medication is given and the rash subsides after 10 days, but the pain diminishes only slightly. For the next few months the patient is plagued by burning and lancinating pain and hyperaesthesia of the affected area. The symptoms are unrelieved by maximum doses of analgesics, including acetaminophen, propoxyphene, ibuprofen, and acetaminophen-codeine combination (Tylenol #3).

On her latest visit to you, the patient is accompanied by her daughter, who says her mother is "acting senile." The daughter explains apologetically that she had read about a "pain clinic" in the local newspaper and took her mother there "out of desperation." At the pain clinic, the patient received a capsule, which she has taken nightly for the past week.

Clue:

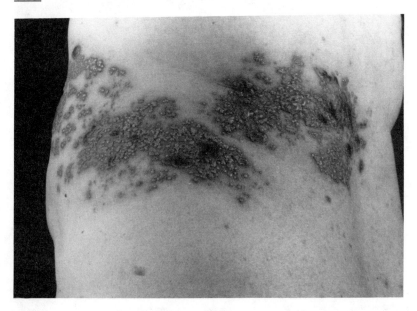

Questions:

1. What initial treatment might have prevented the patient's current pain?

2. What medicine might the patient have received in the pain clinic that caused her confusion?

3. What treatment alternatives exist at this point?

Answers:

1. The patient has recovered from acute cutaneous herpes zoster (shingles) and now has postherpetic neuralgia (PHN), a stubborn problem that affects the elderly more often than the young. A short course of high-dose systemic steroids (40 to 80 mg of prednisone daily for a week, tapered over the next 2 weeks) begun as early as possible in the course of acute shingles may prevent the development of PHN. Oral acyclovir speeds the rate of healing of vesicles and reduces the degree and duration of acute pain in shingles, but has not yet been demonstrated to reduce the incidence of PHN. This may be because treatment is generally not instituted early enough to prevent the nerve damage that is thought to cause the late syndrome. Ideally, steroids and acyclovir should be given during the prodromal (pre-rash) phase, a therapeutic impossibility, since shingles almost always occurs only once.

2. The patient might have received a narcotic analgesic, but in a sophisticated pain clinic tricyclic antidepressants (TCAs) are often given. This patient received doxepin 25 mg nightly. Low doses of TCAs, particularly the strongly serotoninergic agents such as doxepin, imipramine, and amitriptyline, are often effective in alleviating chronic pain sydromes, including certain neuropathies, low back pain, facial pain, and headache. Cancer pain is less likely to respond. The dose required for analgesia is lower than that required for depression, and analgesia generally is obtained with less delay. Unfortunately, the TCAs are not always tolerated by the elderly. This patient developed confusion as a result of the central anticholinergic effect of doxepin. This agent is often selected in the elderly because it is less likely to cause orthostatic hypotension than imipramine or amitriptyline, but it is strongly anticholinergic and not without side effects.

3. Doxepin should be stopped until the confusion subsides. Then an attempt could be made to control the symptoms with a 10-mg dose of doxepin or a less anticholinergic TCA, such as desipramine, although this approach does not necessarily prevent confusion from recurring. Anticonvulsant medication such as phenytoin or carbamazepine may be effective in reducing various forms of neuropathic pain through actions on the axon or synapse, and may be used alone or in combination with a TCA. Nonpharmacologic treatment includes transcutaneous electrical nerve stimulation ("TENS"), ethyl chloride coolant spray followed by rubbing of the affected area, or injection of local anesthetics. Acupuncture and ultrasound have not been found to be effective. In intractable and prolonged cases, nerve block may be helpful. Capsaicin topical analgesic cream (Zostrix) may bring some relief. It is used after herpetic lesions have

healed and is thought to act by depleting substance P, a mediator of pain impulses, from peripheral neurons.

<u>Pearls:</u>

1. The analgesic action of TCAs is thought to be at least partly independent of the antidepressant action, and may be related to their ability to inhibit the enzymatic degradation of enkephalin and to enhance serotonin at the synaptic cleft. Both of these actions are thought to block the pain message as it travels to the central nervous system.

2. The incidence of shingles increases markedly with age. It is thought that the propensity of the elderly to develop shingles is due to the loss of specific cell-mediated immunity to varicella zoster virus (VZV). Although certain malignancies and other immunosuppressive states may predispose to this condition, the development of shingles does not demand a malignancy workup since underlying malignancies are found no more often than in the general population.

3. As many as 50% of untreated patients over the age of 70 have pain for a year or more after the rash has subsided. Symptoms range from severe burning or lancinating pain to itching and tingling. In most cases they diminish over time.

<u>Pitfalls:</u>

1. Although steroids are indicated for the prevention of PHN, they should not be given if shingles has appeared in conjunction with steroid therapy, because continuing or increasing the dose of steroids may convert shingles to generalized zoster.

2. Concentrations of acyclovir required to inactivate VZV are much higher than those required against herpes simplex virus (HSV), and, accordingly, the recommended oral dose used for shingles is 800 mg 5 times a day. Acyclovir is excreted in the kidney and lower doses theoretically should be effective in the elderly, who often have reduced glomerular filtration rate despite normal serum creatinine (see Problem 12, Part II). However, the drug has a very wide therapeutic index when given orally and has been shown to be safe and effective when given at this dose.

3. Involvement of the first division of the trigeminal nerve by VZV can result in severe ocular complications. Acyclovir should be given and ophthalmologic consultation should be obtained immediately to diagnose and manage

potentially serious manifestations such as keratitis and iridocyclitis. Longterm ophthalmologic followup is essential, since possible late effects include glaucoma, cataracts, and blindness.

4. Neurologic complications of shingles are rare, especially in nonimmunocompromised hosts. Patients may develop encephalitis, myelitis, or motor neuropathy with segmental paralysis in the dermatome of the rash. A rare complication of ophthalmic zoster is cerebral angiitis with delayed contralateral hemiplegia. This is thought to be due to viral invasion of cerebral vessels from the contiguous cranial nerve. Despite its rarity, this complication is of interest in geriatric practice because it can be confused with atheroembolic stroke.

References:

Bernstein JE, Bickers DR, Dahl MV, Roshal JY. Treatment of chronic postherpetic neuralgia with topical capsaicin. A preliminary study. J Amer Acad Derm 1987;17:93-96.

Gilbert G. Herpes Zoster ophthalmicus and delayed contralateral hemiparesis. JAMA 1974;229:302-304.

McKendrick MW, MCGill JI, White, JE, Wood MJ. Oral acyclovir in acute herpes zoster. Brit Med J 1986; 293:1529-1532.

Portenoy RK, Duma C, Foley KM. Acute herpetic and postherpetic neuralgia: clinical review and current management. Ann Neurol 1986;20:651-664.

Stauffer JD. Antidepressants and chronic pain. J Fam Practice 1987;25:167-170.

Chronic Cough

<u>Case 3.</u>   An 87-year-old widower, who was living alone in an apartment in a retirement community, complained of a cough productive of scant amounts of greyish sputum for several weeks.   He had no fevers, sweats, or other constitutional symptoms. On physical examination he appeared vigorous and was not coughing. Temperature was 98°F. Auscultation of the lungs revealed scattered rhonchi, which cleared on coughing.   The patient had undergone excision of a malignant melanoma on his back 4 years previously and had been told that "they got it all." He was was a nonsmoker and denied a history of lung disease or exposure to tuberculosis.

Chest x-ray was done and an infiltrate was seen. Sputum culture was sent and a 10-day course of oral ampicillin was instituted.   The cultures were negative and the patient went about his normal business. Six months later he reappeared at the doctor's office complaining of persistent coughing, again without constitutional symptoms. Physical examination was unchanged and the infiltrate was again demonstrated on chest x-ray. The patient now revealed that, "after thinking about it," he remembered that 70 years before, his college roommate had been forced to leave school because of "consumption."

<u>Clue:</u>

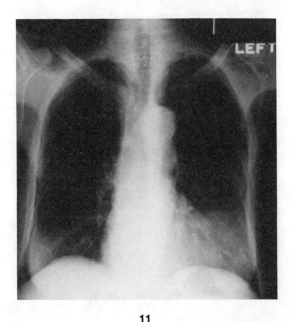

Questions:

1. What further tests are required?

2. Of what diagnostic significance is the chest x-ray?

3. What sequence of events has led to his condition?

4. What preventive medicine efforts should occur at the retirement community?

Answers:

1. Expectorated sputum for gram stain should be done, although a bacterial pneumonia should have made a more definitive statement by this time. The patient has a chronic infiltrate that is most likely due to recurrent melanoma, or to fungal or mycobacterial infection. Sputum for fungal culture and acid fast bacillus should be obtained. If these are negative, chest CT scan should be done, followed by bronchoscopy with cytologic and microbiologic evaluation, and with transbronchial biopsy. Expectorated sputum was positive for M. tuberculosis in this patient.

   Skin test for tuberculosis (TB) should be done because it is simple and safe, but would be more useful in this case if baseline skin test status were known. Although the incidence of positive PPD in asymptomatic American elderly approached 70% fifty years ago, this incidence may be less than 20% today, in parallel with dramatic decline in the incidence of tuberculosis in all age groups. Thus, a positive skin test has more significance today than in previous generations. However, skin test anergy is common in old age, and the incidence of negative PPD in active TB rises with age, so that a negative PPD has limited usefulness in this case as well.

2. Features of the chest x-ray can help distinguish between primary and post-primary (reactivation) tuberculous infection. Positive cultures for TB associated with the isolated lingular infiltrate seen on the patient's x-ray most likely represent primary infection, while lingular infiltrate as an extension of upper lobe disease indicates postprimary disease. Although the vast majority of elderly patients with TB have the reactivation (postprimary) form of the disease, primary infection can occur even in extreme old age, a situation having important epidemiologic significance in the present case.

   The breast shadows seen on the patient's x-ray represent gynecomastia. This had been noted on his physical examination, and is a finding that increases in incidence with age in men. It is unrelated to his present disease.

3. The patient's remote history of TB exposure lends evidence to his having reactivation disease. Reactivation TB may appear to occur spontaneously, but breakdown in the immune system, particularly in T-cell function, is thought to be responsible. The patient has several risk factors. His fairly recent malignancy might have been treated with drugs having immunosuppressant activity, the malignancy might have recurred, or he might have developed a second malignancy. Widowers have been documented in prospective studies to have impaired T-cell function during the time of mourning and have a much higher than expected mortality and rate of illness following death of a spouse. Old age itself brings with it declines in T-cell function, but there is no evidence that age alone predisposes to reactivation of TB. The patient should be

examined carefully for recurrent or second malignancy. Although the diagnosis of primary infection cannot be made with certainty unless the patient's previous skin test reactivity is known, the radiographic picture in this case points to primary infection.

4. Distinguishing primary from postprimary TB becomes important when public health issues are considered. Although the patient has risk factors for reactivation of TB contracted from his college roommate, these same risk factors could have increased his susceptibility to primary TB, to which radiographic evidence points. Interviews, skin testing, and chest x-rays of the patient's contacts should be conducted. If TB skin testing had been required of new residents and employees in the community, retesting at this time would be revealing--it would facilitate discovery of the index case if the patient had primary TB and would identify his contacts at risk for primary disease if he had reactivation TB.

Pearls:

1. TB is three times more common in the elderly population as a whole than in other age groups. TB was very common during youth and young adulthood of the current elder generation, particularly the immigrant population. However, the risk to healthy individuals developing reactivation TB declines significantly with age. The increased risk of developing TB in late life as compared to young adulthood is probably due to the co-occurrence of other risk factors.

2. Negative PPD in active tuberculosis may be due not only to generalized anergy, but also to selective paralysis of a T-cell subset to antigens of M. Tuberculosis.

Pitfalls:

1. Reactivation TB in an elderly patient should not be ascribed to age alone. Most, if not all, cases can be shown to coexist with risk factors such as serious underlying disease, malnutrition, or immunosuppressive treatment.

2. Tuberculosis often presents "atypically" in the elderly, either as "failure to thrive" or as an apparently mild disease without constitutional symptoms. The important thing to keep in mind, however, is that TB can follow the same rules as it does in young adulthood--it is a disease of protean manifestations.

3. The booster phenomenon is more common in the elderly than the young, possibly because of a higher incidence of remote tuberculosis infection or exposure, or remote exposure to nonpathogenic atypical mycobacteria. Elderly patients with negative PPD should be retested within a week in order to distinguish them from individuals who appear to be recent converters on retesting.

References:

American Thoracic Society. The tuberculin skin test. Am Rev Resp Dis 1981;124:356-363.

Khan MA, Kovnat DM, Bachus B, et al. Clinical and roentgenographic spectrum of pulmonary tuberculosis in the adult. Am J Med 1977;62:31-38.

Nagami PH, Yoshikawa TT. Tuberculosis in the elderly geriatric patient. J Am Geriatr Soc 1983;31:356-363.

Schleifer SJ, Keller SE, Camerino M, et al. Suppression of lymphocyte stimulation following bereavement. JAMA 1983;250:374-377.

Stead WW. Tuberculosis among elderly persons: An outbreak in a nursing home. Ann Intern Med 1981;94:606-610.

Stead WW, Lofgren JP, Warren E, et al. Tuberculosis as an endemic and nosocomial infection among the elderly in nursing homes. N Engl J Med 1985;312:1483-1487.

Insomnia (Mrs. B., part 1)

Case 4. A 78-year-old woman is being treated for congestive heart failure, hypothyroidism, recurrent bladder papillomas, atrial fibrillation, osteoarthritis, type II diabetes, and hypertension. She has had a mechanical mitral valve prosthesis for 14 years because of rheumatic heart disease, a history of right cataract excision with a lens implant, and a history of a lower gastrointestinal bleed (colonoscopy revealed diverticuli and an adenomatous polyp). She takes warfarin, digoxin, furosemide, ferrous sulfate, L-thyroxine (Synthroid), acetaminophen, milk of magnesia, methyldopa, and temazepam. You are her new doctor in a busy medical clinic at a large metropolitan hospital. The clinic clerk presents you with three large volumes of her chart. Volume 4 is in urology clinic.

The patient is accompanied by her home attendant. On questioning, the patient admits to shortness of breath, fatigue, urinary frequency, and difficulty sleeping. She is completely alert and able to recite her medication regimen correctly.

Her blood pressure is 130/90, pulse is 60 and irregular. Pertinent findings on her physical examination include obesity, bibasilar rales, holosystolic murmur at the left sternal border, audible valve click, genu varum, and edema of her lower legs. Rectal examination is normal; stool is guaiac negative.

You would like to reevaluate her medications, but you have already spent more than an hour with her, your first of seven patients in your afternoon clinic. You order blood and urine tests and rewrite all of her prescriptions, increasing the furosemide to 60 mg daily.

Laboratory evaluation is unrevealing. Blood sugar is 158 mg/dl. The patient is pleased to find that she no longer requires iron tablets since they make her constipated, and milk of magnesia is discontinued as well. You too are pleased that you no longer have to write seven prescriptions on the complicated hospital form, and while you're at it, you suggest stopping the sleeping medication. She is horrified by the prospect and begs you to write the prescription. When you ask her why she needs the sleeping pill, she gives you a surprised look and says, "I can't sleep." She wakes up at 2 a.m., she says, and can't get back to sleep.

The patient and you establish a good working relationship. Thinking that methyldopa is not good for sleepless, depressed, old women, you are able to taper it without a significant change in her blood pressure, but without a change in her symptoms. She continues to take temazepam nightly.

Six months later on a routine monthly visit, she promptly begins to cry. When asked what's wrong, she says through her tears, "The doctor said I am going to go blind." Volume 4 of her chart is in eye clinic. Volume 3 is missing as well.

Clue:

Amsler's Grid

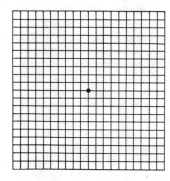

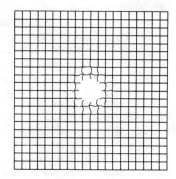

Normal   Image   Patient's   View

Questions:

1. What are the possible factors that could be disturbing her sleep?

2. How is temazepam affecting her sleep? What will happen if you discontinue it?

3. What are the possible things that could be wrong with her vision? What can be done?

4. What questions should you ask this elderly woman to shed light on her insomnia?

Answers:

1. Physiologic changes in sleep occur with age. These include decreases in deep sleep (stages 3 and 4), increased numbers of nocturnal arousals (often unnoticed by the patient), and altered circadian rhythms with a tendency to "phase advance," with sleepiness occurring earlier in the evening and awakening earlier in the morning. Arousals disrupt nocturnal sleep but daytime drowsiness with napping may ensure that total sleep time is not decreased. Many elderly are unable to adjust to altered circadian rhythms and may complain of insomnia, although physiologically they are getting enough sleep.

Disordered sleep in the elderly is often due to such things as depression, fear and worry, nocturia, dyspnea, medication effects, chronic pain syndromes, and ingestion of caffeine or alcohol. All of these factors could be operating in this one patient. Overtreatment with thyroid hormone had to be ruled out (she was found to be euthyroid). Sleep apnea and nocturnal myoclonus disrupt sleep but usually present as daytime drowsiness rather than insomnia. Urinary disturbances are often due to diuretic ingestion and are a cause of noncompliance with this category of medication. Although this patient was pleased with her home attendant, many patients distrust these "strangers," and lie awake with worry, aware that people their age are ideal prey for victimization. Many patients nap during the day and are unable to sleep at night. In such cases, reassurance is called for but may be of no avail.

Patients with dementia are particularly prone to disturbances in normal sleep-wake cycle and are often up at night, agitated, confused, and wandering, but this patient had no evidence of cognitive disturbances.

To find out what Mrs. B.'s problem is, see the answer to question 4.

2. Although tolerance develops more slowly to benzodiazepines than to other hypnotic agents, it does develop. Any help the patient is getting from temazepam at this point is a placebo effect. Abrupt discontinuation of sedative-hypnotics will result in rebound insomnia, and severe withdrawal symptoms may occur if use is long term. All such drugs should be tapered slowly over several weeks. Benzodiazepine receptors are less plastic with age and it may be even more difficult to withdraw these medications in the elderly. Also, patients with chronic insomnia who have been taking sleeping pills for a long time are terribly reluctant to stop. Prior attempts to discontinue medications may have produced rebound insomnia, encouraging prompt resumption of medications. Other patients find that the hypnotic so alters their lifestyle that they are unwilling to go without it. Such patients should nonetheless be cautioned to take the medications intermittently, say, any 3 days of 7. A reluctant prescriber is often viewed as cruel and unsympathetic, and the patient, anxious over the prospect of losing the sleeping pills, might well shop around for a "kind" doctor who "cares about the elderly."

Although the patient has most likely developed tolerance to temazepam, she will probably continue to refuse to do without a sleeping pill, despite the physician's insistence that longterm use of hypnotics is associated with reduced efficacy.   A possible solution to this dilemma is to slowly withdraw the benzodiazepine while instituting nightly tryptophan.   Tryptophan is an amino acid precursor to serotonin and may have sleep-inducing and other effects, particularly when taken chronically.   Since temazepam could no longer be having a hypnotic effect on this patient, an agent devoid of acute effects might prove a good substitute, whether effective or not.

3.   She could well be suffering from decreasing visual acuity from a left cataract, a process accelerated by the presence of diabetes.   Like most patients with mild type II diabetes, however, she did not have diabetic retinopathy of the proliferative variety, nor did she have background retinopathy that is more commonly seen.   Due to her frequent visits to ophthalmologists, she has had adequate screening for chronic open angle glaucoma, and this has been ruled out.   Open angle glaucoma is "silent" until visual loss is severe, since peripheral vision is lost first while central vision is maintained.   This patient has macular degeneration, affecting her central vision.   Macular degeneration is the most common cause of legal blindness (corrected visual acuity of 20/200 or worse) in the elderly.   The Amsler's grid, when viewed by the patient, will appear distorted in places, or portions will disappear, particularly in the field of central vision.

Once low vision has been established, counseling and rehabilitation are mandatory.   Often the elderly are left with the impression that "nothing can be done."   The patient's ophthalmologist could refer the patient for low vision evaluation and rehabilitation.   The National Center for Low Vision in New York City maintains a directory of low vision centers around the country, and can be contacted if further information is required.

4.   It is very important to ask the right question when evaluating a sleep disorder.   What are her sleep patterns?   Does she sleep during the day?   Does she consume alcohol, caffeine, or over-the-counter pills or eye drops that can disrupt sleep?   Is she awakened by shortness of breath?   Need to urinate?   The physician did not ask what time she was going to bed.   She was in fact bedding down at 8 o'clock, and sometimes fell asleep quite readily, sleeping until 2 a.m.   Tolerance to temazepam has most certainly developed, causing counterproductive disordered sleep.   This particular patient went to bed out of boredom. Her friends and family were either dead or inaccessible; there was danger in going out after dark to visit what friends she had, the elderly commonly being victims of muggings and purse snatchings.   She suffered from low vision and was unable to watch television, read, or sew.   As a result, she had nothing to do in the evening but sleep.   She claimed not to have been

awakened by the need to urinate, a common cause of disordered sleep even in normal elderly whose urinary cycle may have taken a circadian turn (as had her sleep cycle). Furosemide is normally a short-acting agent but its duration of action may be prolonged in the elderly and may cause urinary symptoms longer than expected. Nocturia is often a reason why elderly patients fail to comply with diuretic therapy. This patient's denial of the problem should prompt the physician to question whether the patient is taking her full dose.

Pearls:

1. There are two kinds of macular degeneration--"dry" (atrophic) and "wet" (exudative, disciform). "Dry" macular degeneration is associated with atrophy of retinal pigment epithelium and may lead to slowly progressive loss of central vision. In the exudative variety, loss of central vision can be profound and sometimes occurs suddenly. Oozing of delicate subretinal vessels can cause a disciform avascular scar that promotes the formation of neovasculature, friable vessels that are prone to rupture. When macular degeneration results in legal blindness, up to 90% of the time it is in the 10% of patients with this more serious form of the disease.

Further hemorrhage, damage, and loss of visual acuity can be prevented by laser photocoagulation of neovasculature. Although there is no known preventive maneuver for atrophic macular degeneration, the patient has much more time to adjust to the slow loss of vision. Peripheral vision is preserved and optical aids can enhance central vision. The present patient had this form of the disease and had a probable life expectancy much shorter than her visual life.

2. Temazepam is actually the benzodiazepine hypnotic of choice in the elderly because it is metabolized to inactive metabolites, does not accumulate over time, and has an intermediate duration of action that minimizes next-day sedation. As a benzodiazepine, it probably does not participate in any significant drug-drug interactions. This is particularly important in patients taking warfarin, with which several nonbenzodiazepine hypnotics interact. Temazepam does, however, have a delayed onset of action in its hard capsule form, and should be given at least 1 hour before bedtime.

3. Although benzodiazepines are highly bound to serum proteins, they do not appear to displace coumadin from its binding sites, presumably because these agents are bound at different sites.

Pitfalls:

1. Flurazepam is an excellent benzodiazepine hypnotic agent, having a rapid onset of action, but it is degraded in the liver by Phase I (oxidative) processes to an active metabolite with an ultra-long half-life. Phase I metabolism is sluggish in the elderly, so that the overall elimination half-life of flurazepam may be as long as 300 hours in some patients. Temazepam undergoes Phase II metabolism (conjugation), the rate of which is unchanged with age.

2. Triazolam is a potent benzodiazepine with a rapid onset and short duration of action, does not accumulate, has a low tendency to cause next-day sedation, and, when taken judiciously, causes restful sleep and may even improve daytime performance. Despite these potential advantages for the geriatric patient, however, it is not the hypnotic of first choice. Its short duration lends itself to seemingly paradoxical reactions that actually represent acute withdrawal syndromes. It is probably more likely to cause delirium and retrograde amnesia in the elderly than other agents. If used, the starting dose should be 0.125 mg or less.

3. Certain sedating antihistamines are often used as hypnotics because they are considered "mild" and are nonaddicting. The problem is that tolerance to the sedative effects develops fairly soon, but tolerance may not develop to its anticholinergic effects. These agents are available over-the-counter and patients may self-administer increasing doses to obtain sleep. In such cases, elderly patients easily develop anticholinergic side effects such as constipation, confusion, blurred vision, urinary retention, and dry mouth. Caution is required.

References:

Ferris FL. Senile macular degeneration: review of epidemiologic features. Am J Epidemiol 1983;118:132-151.

Greenblatt DJ, Shader RI, Abernethy DR. Current status of benzodiazepines. N Engl J Med 1983;309:354-358, 410-416.

Howard GF. Management of chronic sleep disorders in the elderly. Comp Ther 1987;13:3-9.

National Institute of Mental Health, Drugs and Insomnia: The use of medications to promote sleep. JAMA 1984;251:2410-2414.

Pressman MR, Fry JM. What is normal sleep in the elderly? Clin Geriatr Med 1988;4:71-81.

Roth T, Roehrs TA (eds). Sleep disorders in the elderly. Clin Geriatr Med 1989;5(2).

Schneider-Helmert D, Spinweber CL. Evaluation of L-tryptophan for treatment of insomnia: a review. Psychopharmacol 1986;89:1-7.

Weakness (Mrs. B., part 2)

<u>Case 5.</u> Mrs. B. asks to see you because of weakness. She is pale. Her blood pressure is 120/80. Her heart rate is 100 and irregular. Hematocrit is 24%. On her last visit to you 6 weeks ago, methyldopa was replaced with hydralazine (Apresoline). Her prescribed regimen now is:

Warfarin (Coumadin) 5 mg or 7.5 mg on alternate days
Digoxin 0.125 mg every other day
L-Thyroxine (Synthroid) 100 μg plus 25 μg daily
Furosemide 40 mg every morning, 20 mg afternoons
Apresoline 10 mg t.i.d.
Acetaminophen as needed for arthritic pain
Temazepam 15 mg as needed for sleep

Volume 4 of her hospital chart is in urology clinic.

Clue:

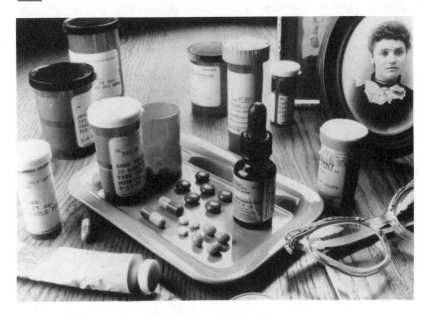

Questions:

1. How might the patient's drug regimen have resulted in a drop in hematocrit?

2. What tests should be done?

3. How did her problem occur?

4. How can compliance be improved?

5. Describe four pharmacokinetic changes that occur with age.

Answers:

1. A complicated medical regimen can be impossible to adhere to, and life-threatening problems can occur.   Compliance with any medical regimen is inversely proportional to the number of pills prescribed, unless the disease is producing symptoms. Astoundingly, this patient is able to recite her prescribed regimen accurately, although this does not guarantee that she is taking it accurately.   Of importance at the moment is whether the patient is "overcoumadinized."

2. Prothrombin time (PT) and stool guaiac must be done. Her PT had been 1.3 times control but was now much higher, and resulted in a gastrointestinal bleed. Platelet count was normal. Endoscopic evaluation was done to see if a discrete lesion was present. Coombs' test is also an important part of the evaluation, since another possible drug-related cause of anemia is Coombs-positive hemolysis due to methyldopa, which she had been taking as recently as 4 weeks before. Methyldopa-related anemia occurs in a delayed fashion, weeks to months after the drug is instituted. Autoimmune hemolytic anemia is thought to occur more commonly in the elderly because of age-related impairment in T-cell function, in this case of the suppressor cell subset, but another factor could be the greater drug use in the elderly. Her Coombs' test was negative.

Hydralazine-induced lupus-like reaction can produce anemia, but a positive antinuclear antibody reaction must be interpreted with caution because of the high incidence of harmless, low-titer autoantibodies found in well elderly.

3. Incorrect administration of the drug regimen must be assumed until proven otherwise. Visual disorders exacerbate the problem of compliance, since many pills look alike. Coumadin, Apresoline, and Synthroid resemble one another, as do a multitude of other drugs, and one of the many possible errors could have been that the patient took three Coumadin tablets instead of three Apresoline.

The usual cause of increased sensitivity to warfarin is a drug-drug interaction. A meticulous drug history should be done to see if new drugs, including over-the-counter agents, have been introduced since her last visit. This patient visited the urologist one week before and was treated for a urinary tract infection with trimethoprim-sulfamethoxazole (Bactrim). Sulfa drugs, like an array of other agents, interact with warfarin, in this case, by displacing the anticoagulant from protein-binding sites and increasing the free (active) fraction of the drug.

4. It is important to observe elderly patients open the bottles and demonstrate the regimen.   Pills should be in containers that the patient can open.

Envelopes can be substituted for bottles if necessary. Instructions should be written legibly on container labels or on a medication instruction card. It is important to ascertain if the patient can read. Mrs. B. came from Poland and never learned to read English. Facility in the language of the adopted country is often not attained by elderly immigrants. Mrs. B's illiteracy was discovered late in her doctor's acquaintance with her, and, because of good home care, did not create a problem.

Compliance can be facilitated with the use of medication-reminder boxes, available at most drug stores, which the patient or a caregiver can prefill weekly, although these devices may not help cognitively impaired patients.

Patients should always be instructed to consult the primary care physician before taking any new medication prescribed by another physician or purchased over-the-counter.

The medication regimen must be simplified! If budget allows, the patient should purchase a 125 μg Synthroid tablet. Need for digoxin should be re-evaluated since her dose is quite small. Furosemide can be given as a once-daily dose if it is being used for an edematous state. Once hematocrit normalizes, the need for antihypertensive treatment should be reevaluated. If treatment is needed, a once-daily agent such as enalapril should be considered, or, because of age-related pharmacokinetic changes, the patient could have a trial of a multiple-dose agent fewer times a day, such as once-daily clonidine or twice-daily diltiazem. Warfarin, of course, must be given exactly as PT dictates, but in patients at high risk of adverse effects, it should not be given unless there is an absolute indication.

There are many reasons to discontinue hypnotics ("Mrs. B., Part 1"), but most people refuse to discontinue them. In any case, hypnotics are pills that few people forget to take.

5.   a. Renal function declines with age, on the average, delaying clearance of renally excreted drugs such as digoxin.

b. "Phase I" hepatic metabolism (oxidation-reduction) declines with age, so that drugs handled by these processes may be metabolized more slowly, all other factors being equal. "Phase II" metabolism remains intact. This group of reactions involves attachment of the drug to a larger endogenous molecule (e.g., glucuronidation and acetylation), producing generally inactive, renally excreted metabolites. Thus, temazepam, which is metabolized by glucuronidation, is metabolized readily and dose adjustments may not be necessary, while its close relative diazepam is metabolized by oxidation with resulting prolonged elimination half-life in the elderly, requiring that caution be used in prescribing. The Phase I-Phase II schema is useful but not an accurate predictor of drug dosing because of the multiplicity of factors involved in drug handling. Thus, warfarin, which undergoes Phase I metabolism, does not seem to have a reduced elimination half-life because of other pharmacokinetic variables, but lower doses are required for the elderly to produce the same blood level seen in younger subjects on higher doses, which may be due to such age-related influences as impaired vitamin K status or reduced clotting factor precursors.

    c. Levels of serum proteins are often depressed in sick elderly. This increases the free fraction of highly bound drugs, such as warfarin, but free drug can reach organs of metabolism and excretion more readily, so that equilibrium is reached and the effect may not be clinically significant on a chronic basis.

    d. Total body fat increases and lean body mass decreases with age as the percentage of total body weight. Therefore, the volume of distribution (V_D) of lipid-soluble drugs increases with age, while the V_D of water-soluble drugs decreases with age. Simplistically speaking, lipid-soluble drugs such as diazepam and its metabolites tend to accumulate in tissues, resulting in delayed toxicity, while water-soluble drugs, such as alcohol, have a higher peak plasma level after a given initial dose, and may produce an exaggerated response.

Pearls:

1. The therapeutic range of PT considered to be optimal for anticoagulation, once considered to be up to 2.5 times the control value, has been revised downward to a level at which adequate anticoagulation can be achieved with a lower risk of bleeding. Prior guidelines were developed when a less sensitive PT was used. The older thromboplastin reagent was more responsive to warfarin-induced reductions in vitamin-K-dependent factors, producing prolongation of PT on a lower dose of warfarin than would be needed using reagents in general use today. Unfortunately, this revision has not yet caught on, and many physicians are still using the older guidelines. In most cases, adequate anticoagulation can be achieved when PT is held at 1.3 times the control. This is particularly important for the elderly, who, as a group, are at high risk of bleeding.

2. Dose-adjustments should be considered for renally excreted drugs. This is particularly important when there is a narrow therapeutic-to-toxic ratio, as in the case of digoxin or gentamicin, and less important for ordinary doses of less toxic agents like furosemide or penicillin.

3. Pharmacodynamic factors may be at least as important as pharmacokinetic ones. Thyroid hormone is not only cleared more slowly, but is more likely to produce cardiac effects in older patients, who often have heart disease.

Pitfalls:

1. The elderly experience a greater number of bleeding episodes from warfarin than do younger adults. Assuming that PT is held within an acceptable therapeutic range, the increased danger is probably the result of drug-drug interactions and the presence of underlying bleedable lesions.

2. Ultra-long acting agents such as flurazepam, piroxecam, and chlorpropamide must be used cautiously in the elderly since their duration of action may be even longer than desired. It is often better to try an intermediate or semi-long acting agent on a once-a-day basis first, when the convenience of once-a-day dosing is desired.

3. Generic formulations have less distinctive markings than do brand-name drugs, and when changes in brand are made at the drug store, the physician is hardly ever aware. One patient with low vision had been taking Cardizem (diltiazem) 60 mg and Inderal (propranolol) 80 mg. She decided to save money by purchasing generic propranolol, but the new drug so closely resembled diltiazem that she could not tell them apart.

4. Serum creatinine does not accurately reflect decreases in glomerular filtration rate late in life because muscle mass, the source of measured creatinine, declines with age (see Problem 12, Part II).

References:

Alberts MJ, Massey W, Dawson D. A multicenter study of anticoagulation parameters when using heparin and warfarin. Arch Neurol 1987;44:1229-1231.

American College of Chest Physicians and the National Heart, Lung, and Blood Institute. National conference on antithrombotic therapy. Chest 1986;2 (Supp):1s-106s.

Greenblatt DJ, Sellers EM, Shader RI. Drug disposition in old age. N Engl J Med 1982;306:1081-1088.

Hulka BS, Kupper LL, Cassel JC, Efird RL. Medication use and misuse: physician-patient discrepancies. J Chron Dis 1975;28:7-21.

Lamy PP. Over-the-counter medication: the drug interactions we overlook. J Am Geriatr Soc 1982;30(Supp):S67-S75.

Petz LD. Drug-induced hemolytic anemia. Clin Hematol 1980;9:455-482.

Vaginal Bleeding

<u>Case 6.</u>   An 88-year-old woman with advanced Alzheimer's dementia has been residing in a nursing home for 2 years.   She does not speak, is incontinent, and cannot feed herself.   Her internal organs seem to be functioning admirably and she receives no medication except for a "bowel regimen" that consists of a stool softener, milk of magnesia, and occasional tap water enemas.

One day the nurse notices blood on the patient's incontinence pants (adult diapers) and reports to the physician that the patient has vaginal bleeding.

Clue:

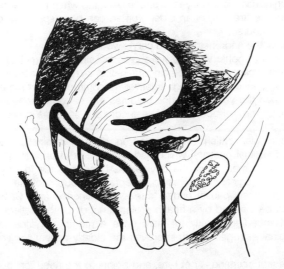

Adapted from Davis CH, ed. Gynecology and obstetrics. Hagerstown MD: WF Prior Co, Inc, 1933.

Questions:

1. What is the best way to confirm the presence of vaginal bleeding?

2. What are common causes of postmenopausal bleeding?

3. How can this patient's problem be handled?

Answers:

1. Since blood stains can indicate bleeding from the gastrointestinal or urinary tract, a bimanual examination of the vagina should be performed. Insertion of a tampon into the patient's vagina can also confirm whether the suspected site is, indeed, vaginal.

2. Vaginal bleeding in elderly women is most often due to atrophic vaginitis, endometrial hyperplasia, or gynecologic malignancies. Endometrial hyperplasia is more common in women who have taken postmenopausal estrogens, but occasionally is due to endogenous estrogen production by an ovarian tumor. Atrophic vaginitis is more likely to produce bleeding when there is trauma to the mucosa, but the "trauma" in an older woman can be a speculum examination or sexual intercourse.

Cancer of the endometrium and cervix would have to be considered in this patient, even if atrophic vaginitis were present, since endometrial cancer and invasive cervical cancer (unlike carcinoma-in-situ) increase in incidence with age. Vulvar and vaginal cancer, though relatively uncommon, affect the elderly more commonly than the young. Uterine myomas are estrogen sensitive and tend to regress after the menopause, but the uncommon sarcoma generally presents later in life.

This particular patient was found, on digital examination, to have an incarcerated vaginal pessary, which had been inserted prior to her admission to the nursing home. Thus, the device has been in place for 2 years at the very least. The vaginal pessary is an acceptable (though not the only) method of treating postmenopausal urinary stress incontinence (see Case 16). The pessary can be inserted by a health professional or by the patient herself, but must be changed frequently (at least once a month), or incarceration may result. Vaginal estrogen cream improves the elderly patient's tolerance of the pessary.

The present scenario is not rare, and points to the need for routine vaginal examination of women upon admission to a longterm care facility.

3. Often, an incarcerated pessary can be removed manually without complications, but if it does not come out readily, topical estrogen treatment for a few days may facilitate removal. Surgical intervention is usually not required.

The approach to vaginal bleeding in profoundly demented patients like the present one should be handled on an individual basis. Physical examination is a must, but extensive workup is usually not warranted.

Pearl:

Elderly patients with dementia of the Alzheimer type have been thought, in general, to be otherwise healthier than age-matched patients without Alzheimer's disease. This common clinical bias has recently been reported in a controlled study. The reasons for this finding are not known and may simply reflect the fact that healthy patients survive long enough to develop this late-onset disease. Alternatively, it may illustrate how every human being eventually develops at least one disease and the law of averages sets limits on the number of diseases suffered by most people.

Pitfalls:

1. Bedridden patients with advanced Alzheimer's disease and other debilitating neurologic diseases may develop flexion contractures of the hips unless bedside range-of-motion exercises are given regularly. These deformities can severely limit the pelvic examination.

2. Vulvar excoriations may also cause genital bleeding in elderly demented patients, especially in the presence of vulvar dystrophies ("leukoplakia," and other epithelial lesions). Severely debilitated patients are often treated with "benign neglect," and care as seemingly mundane as nail cutting may be omitted. Neglected fingernails may also produce skin irritation, infection in the digits, and impaired manual dexterity. (Neglected toenails, in addition, can adversely affect ambulation.)

References:

Poma PA. Management of incarcerated vaginal pessaries. J Am Geriatr Soc 1981;29:325-327.

Rubin SC. Postmenopausal bleeding: etiology, evaluation, and management. Med Clin N Amer 1987;71:59-69.

Wolf-Klein GP, Silverstone FA, Brod MS, et al. Are Alzheimer patients healthier? J Am Geriatr Soc 1988;36:219-224.

Reversible Dementia

<u>Case 7.</u>   A 79-year-old woman is admitted to the surgical service of a community hospital because of an acute abdomen.

The patient is a mild diabetic controlled on diet but had been in apparently good physical condition until 3 days prior to admission when she developed abdominal pain.   The patient had not complained of inability to move her bowels, although, according to the patient's husband, she has "always been constipated," and had taken laxatives "for years." He also notes that she had deteriorated mentally in her past year or so, becoming forgetful and unable to manage her personal needs.   Recently, she has become incontinent of urine. Family and friends feel that she is "getting senile."

On physican examination, she is lethargic.   Her pulse is 56 and regular. Temperature is 97.2°F.   Abdomen is slightly distended and diffusely tender. Neurologic examination is normal except for depressed deep tendon reflexes. White blood count is 11,000 with a normal differential; blood glucose is 160 mg/dL. She is treated with hydration and enemas, her abdominal symptoms resolve, and her lethargy clears.   White count returns to normal.   She is discharged to a teaching nursing home.   Discharge diagnoses are fecal impaction and "O.B.S."

She is admitted to a nursing home where screening laboratory tests are done and one result indicates that her dementia may be due to a reversible disease. A closer look at the patient reveals a pertinent physical finding.

<u>Clue:</u>

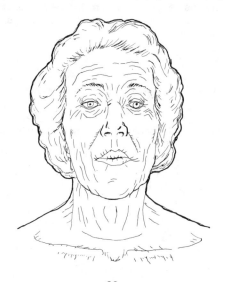

32

Questions:

1. What key blood test was not done by the surgeons?

2. The underlying cause of dementia is treated. What changes, if any, might occur in the patient's:

    a. mental status?
    b. bowel habits?
    c. cardiac status?
    d. diabetes?
    e. urinary symptoms?

3. What caution should the treating physician observe?

Answers:

1. The surgeons had an abdominal emergency on their hands and did not consider the possibility that the patient's subacute mental decline could be reversible. The usual automated chemistries quickly check for many causes of reversible confusion, but most do not include thyroid function tests. Because hypothyroidism is usually subtle or occult in the elderly, and the prevalence is high, many geriatricians perform thyroid function tests routinely on all new patients. The screening test selected in the nursing home was a total T_4 level, with follow-up T_3 resin uptake or TSH done as indicated. The patient's T_4 was 0.6 μg/dL (N = 6.2-13.2) and her TSH was 90 μU/mL (N = 0.8-4.8).

The patient was found to have a faint thyroidectomy scar on her neck that had not been previously noticed. An old scar can be as difficult to spot on a patient, if you are not looking for one, as it is to detect on the illustration. Thyroidectomy is only one cause of hypothyroidism in the elderly.

Serum vitamin B_{12} should be done on elderly patients with undiagnosed dementia or new affective disorders, since B_{12} deficiency can cause neurologic damage even in the absence of anemia. It is not generally recommended as a screening test because of its low specificity.

2. a.   Treatment of severe hypothyroidism in this patient resulted in almost complete resolution of her dementia. Demented patients with modest hypothyroidism usually do not improve because the dementia is coincidental and of another cause.

   b.   Constipation improved slightly. Improvement is not guaranteed in chronically constipated elderly who have the problem on another basis, in this case, possible laxative abuse.

   c.   Bradycardia resolved with treatment. This also is not guaranteed in geriatric practice where underlying sick sinus syndrome is common.

   d.   The patient's blood sugar increased with treatment. Thyroid hormone may worsen glucose tolerance in diabetics by increasing absorption of dietary carbohydrates and by increasing metabolic clearance of endogenous insulin.

   e.   Urinary incontinence was due to the patient's confusion. With the resolution of the confusional state, the patient toileted herself appropriately.

3. Treatment of this patient's hypothyroidism is urgent but not emergent, since she is not in myxedema coma. Because the elderly often have underlying cardiac disease, the starting dose of thyroxine should be low (generally 25 micrograms per day) and should be increased by no more than 25 microgram

increments every 3 to 4 weeks, until TSH is near normal (normalization of TSH may lag behind actual repletion of thyroid hormone). Since silent ischemia is common in both elderly and diabetics, periodic EKG should be done. This patient developed asymptomatic T-wave inversions during her treatment and thyroid replacement had to be slowed.

Pearls:

1. The combination of normal thyroxine levels and modestly elevated TSH is referred to as the "failing thyroid syndrome," and is common in the elderly. Some experts feel this should be treated to prevent overt hypothyroidism. Others disagree.   Since most elderly patients with this syndrome are asymptomatic or have nonspecific symptoms that look hypothyroid (constipation, confusion, dry skin) but are not, and that do not resolve with treatment, it is probably sensible to follow these patients by measuring TSH levels every 6 to 8 months, and telling them to contact the physician if they feel ill.

2. Many elderly patients with hypothyroidism have no prior history of overt thyroid disease. Pathological examination of thyroid glands reveals atrophy and "burned-out" thyroiditis. This patient's history was remote, and remained a mystery.

Pitfalls:

1. Although as many as 20% of dementia cases are reversible, longstanding dementia in patients over age 75, which has been of insidious onset, usually is due to Alzheimer's disease.   On close questioning the family will acknowledge that clues of cognitive decline were present for several years. Because of recent publicity about dementia, family members often make pilgrimages to geriatricians for third and fourth opinions. The present case represents an unusual but happy outcome, in which "senility" was assumed but metabolic disease was discovered. Of note is the fact that the course was subacute, possibly less than 1 year.

2. In the elderly, symptoms of hypothyroidism, such as constipation, bradycardia, confusion, dry skin, fatigue, and coarse voice, are utterly nonspecific. Although the presence of one or more of these symptoms should prompt a laboratory investigation, the patient is more often found to be euthyroid than hypothyroid, and sometimes is found to be hyperthyroid.

References:

Gambert SR, Tsitouras PD. Effect of age on thyroid hormone physiology and function. J Am Geriatr Soc 1985;33:360-365.

Hodkinson HM, Irvine RE. The endocrine system--thyroid disease in the elderly. In: Brocklehurst JC, Textbook of geriatric medicine and gerontology. 3rd ed. Edinburgh: Churchill Livingstone, 1985:686-714.

Horowitz, GR. What is a complete work-up for dementia? Clin Geriatr Med 1988;4:163-180.

Progressive Dementia

Case 8: An 80-year-old woman was admitted to a hospital because of fever and intractable decubitus ulcers.

The patient had been in excellent health until approximately 9 years before when her family began to notice that she was getting forgetful. Over the years, her memory slowly worsened, and her previously immaculate grooming was replaced by a disheveled appearance that included stained clothes and unmatched shoes. She sometimes exhibited paranoid behavior, accusing her husband of having an affair with her devoted friend Arlene, who visited often.

As her intellect continued to decline, the patient occasionally became very depressed. Words often failed her, although her speech was fluent. Her husband complained that she behaved like "an infant," tearing books that she once read avidly, pouring coffee into the sugar cannister, and nibbling from several different pieces of fruit in one fruit bowl. She began to walk with a stooped posture, became incontinent of urine and feces, and was admitted to a nursing home, where she eventually became bedridden, contracted, and mute, requiring total care.

She was admitted to a hospital twice because of aspiration pneumonia, and eventually developed decubitus ulcers over her greater trochanter and ischial tuberosity, which penetrated to bone. When fever developed she was again admitted to the hospital, where she was treated with intravenous antibiotics. The decubitus ulcers were treated with cleansing, debridement, and dressing changes, but did not resolve, and if antibiotics were stopped, fever and bacteremia resumed. During the prolonged hospitalization, the patient's husband received a bill from the hospital for nearly $30,000, demanding immediate payment. Already depressed over his wife's illness, he now became despondent, fearing rapid depletion of his life savings. A family member called the hospital in protest, but was told that the patient's "lifetime Medicare days have been used up." A hospital lawyer suggested that the husband divorce his wife in order to protect his savings, but at the mere mention of the word "divorce," the husband became enraged, exclaiming, "We have been married for 50 years! How can I divorce her now?"

The patient was visited frequently by her family and her friend, Arlene. A former psychologist, who held a doctorate degree, the patient had often expressed dismay over living with "less than a brain," having once told Arlene that "if anything like that [dementia] ever happens to me, tell them to shoot me." It is Arlene who now gently suggests to the family that "perhaps treatment should stop."

Clue:

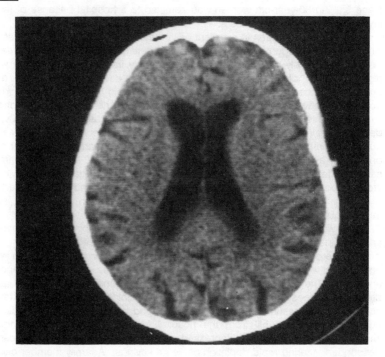

Questions:

1. What disease has caused the patient's underlying dementia? How do you know?

2. What treatment can be offered for the dementia?

3. What is the cause of this disease? What are the risk factors?

4. Is the patient's husband responsible for the hospital bill?

5. Is it permissible for antibiotics to be withheld, even if the outcome is certain death?

Answers:

1. The patient's clinical course is consistent with Alzheimer's disease (AD). There is simply no other disease affecting the elderly that has this type of slowly progressive course consisting of gradual loss of memory and higher intellectual function. Variations in presentation have been reported, including predominance of aphasia, apraxia, or agnosia, or the presence of extrapyramidal signs, but neuropathological confirmation does not always accompany these reports. In the late stages of AD, the patient becomes immobile and often develops contractions, cannot speak, and may lose the ability to swallow.

The diagnosis of AD is a clinical one that relies on history, mental status testing, absence of "hard" neurologic findings, and exclusion of other forms of dementia. Other causes of dementia should be ruled out by laboratory evaluation but it should be emphasized that, when other diseases are found in the midst of the syndrome described in this patient, they are usually superimposed on AD. This approach at best leads to a diagnosis of "probable AD," for currently, AD can be definitively diagnosed only with brain biopsy, which would be inappropriate in all but a few cases.

Neuroimaging techniques such as computed tomography (CT) and magnetic resonance imaging reveal cortical atrophy and are employed to rule out other structural causes of cognitive impairment. Currently used techniques are not sensitive enough to distinguish between atrophy of AD and age-related cortical atrophy seen in normal elderly. Positron emission tomography (PET) scanning shows regional areas of decreased glucose uptake, the extent of which correlates with the severity of dementia, but PET remains a research tool. Specific serologic markers are being sought but are not in use at this time. This patient underwent CT scanning, which revealed "moderate cortical atrophy consistent with patient age."

Pick's disease is a rare cause of progressive dementia that may be confused with AD. Pathologically, there is a disproportionate atrophy of the frontal and temporal lobes, and histologic features are quite different from AD. Clinically, PD may have a more variable presentation than AD, and is said to be characterized by a predominance of "frontal lobe" symptoms, such as apathy, but the rarity of PD has prevented its precise characterization. The etiology is not known. Differentiation from AD is not crucial, since treatment is the same.

2. There is no specific treatment that reverses the dementia. However, this does not mean that "nothing can be done." Any superimposed illness that can reversibly worsen cognition (e.g., infection, drugs, metabolic disease) should be sought and treated, if doing so will return the patient to a more functional state. Some investigators recommend the use of ergoloid mesylates

(Hydergine) in the early stages of dementia. This agent probably has a nonspecific mood-altering effect and cannot be considered a major treatment modality, but its popularity derives from its lack of side effects and the family's urging for some assistance.

In a patient such as the present one, who has end-stage AD, treatment should focus on comfort care, family counseling, and investigation of the patient's previously expressed wishes or life's philosophy with regard to treatment of terminal illness. If the patient is living at home, the family must be made aware of the array of social services for personal and financial counseling and home care, and the availability of self-help groups such as the Alzheimer's Disease Association.

3. The cause of AD is not known, but at least in some cases is thought to have a strong genetic component, inherited in an autosomal dominant pattern, and expressed in a delayed onset, making family history a risk factor. Advanced age is a major risk factor. Less is known about extrinsic factors such as toxins, history of head trauma, or infection with atypical agents such as prion or slow virus, but these and other etiologies are under investigation.

4. In most states, under current Medicare regulations, married people are responsible for each other's medical bills. Medicare law and its interpretations are constantly changing, however, and recent developments have allowed spouses in some localities to keep their savings if they can demonstrate that their health requires such protection. In many cases, "healthy" spouses have divorced sick ones in order to protect their savings. In the present case, which took place a few years ago, an attorney specializing in Medicare law was consulted and cited a recent minor change in the law that recalculated her 100 "lifetime" Medicare days: she had spent sufficient time in a nursing home receiving only custodial care between hospitalizations, and the first day of her most recent hospitalization now counted as day 1.

As of the writing of this book, a Federal "catastrophic health care law" has extended Medicare coverage greatly for hospitalization, but modestly for nursing home care. There is still no Medicare coverage for custodial longterm care. The law does promise to offer partial income protection to the "healthy" spouse of nursing home residents.

This case illustrates the mind-boggling complexity of reimbursement. Most elderly and their spouses do not have the awareness, will, energy, or financial resources to fight such battles.

5. It is permissible for antibiotics to be withheld in this case, because it is in compliance with what the patient would have wished (see Case 9). Decisions to forego medical care should be made after close consultation with family members or other involved parties who can reasonably be ascertained to be

acting in the patient's best interests.   Like most elderly, this patient did not have a Living Will, but her wishes were inferred from her life's philosophy about which she had once been quite vocal.   In order to further ensure that extraordinary measures are not taken to keep this patient alive against her wishes in case of a cardiac or respiratory arrest, a do-not-resuscitate (DNR) order should be written in accordance with current guidelines of the Joint Commission on Accreditation of Healthcare Organizations, and local regulations.

Pearls:

1.   AD was first described in 1906 in a 55-year-old woman, and for many years was referred to as "presenile dementia," to be distinguished from senile dementia ("senility"), which was attributed to "hardening of the arteries." Extensive autopsy study in the 1960's revealed that the majority of elderly dements have the brain histopathology of classic AD, although many have evidence of vascular etiology as well.   The medical community and the public are only now accepting the equivalence of "senility" and AD.

2.   By age 35, all patients with Down's syndrome have histopathological and neurochemical changes in their brains identical with AD.   Also, the incidence of Down's syndrome is higher in families of patients with AD than in the general population.   These observations have led to the discovery of an AD-associated gene on the long arm of chromosome 21.   This site is near the region associated with Down's syndrome and near the gene coding for a precursor to brain amyloid found in AD.   Amyloid is thought by some to be important in the pathophysiology of AD, but much work needs to be done to elucidate the association.

3.   Patients with AD often exhibit "primitive reflexes," such as grasp, snout, and palmomental.   These are thought to be due to deterioration in cortical inhibitory centers that ablate these reflexes after infancy.   In the later stages of AD, posture becomes stooped, and the patient eventually assumes the "fetal position."   Primitive reflexes are a nonspecific finding, being seen in a significant minority of clinically normal elderly.

Pitfalls:

1.   The presence of paranoia in AD does not necessarily indicate an additional psychiatric disease.   In AD, paranoid symptoms may be secondary to memory loss.   The patient forgot who her friend was and assumed it was a mistress. Another patient misplaced expensive jewelry and insisted that people were stealing from her.   Paranoid delusions are common in this setting, however, and may be related to underlying organic brain disease.   Persistent paranoid

delusions may produce harmful or disruptive behavior, which can be managed with low doses of neuroleptics such as thioridazine or haloperidol.

2. A common cause of progressive dementia in the elderly is so-called "multi-infarct dementia" (MID). The classic syndrome is that of a stepwise decline in cognition due to disease in small, perforating arteries, which results in an accumulation of lacunar strokes. MID often coexists with AD. Treatment consists of reducing risk factors for stroke, but since no good study has shown this to be effective, invasive procedures such as carotid arteriography are usually not warranted. The vascular disease seen in some cases of the broad category of MID may have a different etiology than classic cerebrovascular disease.

3. Protections of patient autonomy do not extend to the patient's apparent belief in active euthanasia. "Active euthanasia" implies the taking of positive action that causes a patient to die. Although American courts have tended to be lenient in a few cases of known active euthanasia by family members of hopelessly ill patients, this remains illegal. Active euthanasia is openly practiced in Holland under strict professional guidelines, but, contrary to popular belief, is illegal in that country as well.

The term "passive euthanasia," is often used to refer to the process of allowing incurable illness to produce death by withholding or withdrawing treatment. If this is in compliance with the patient's wishes, it is considered acceptable medical practice.

References:

Basavaraju NG, Silverstone FA, Libow LS, et al. Primitive reflexes and perceptual sensory tests in the elderly--their usefulness in dementia. J Chron Dis 1981;34:367-377.

Besdine RW. Dementia and delirium. In: Rowe JW, Besdine RW. Geriatric medicine. 2nd ed. Boston: Little, Brown, 1988:375-401.

Blessed G, Tomlinson BE, Roth M. The association between quantitative measures of dementia and of senile change in the cerebral grey matter of elderly subjects. Brit J Psychiatr 1968;114:797-811.

Butler RN. "Catastrophic coverage": Good, but we can do better. Geriatrics 1988;43(8):11,14.

Hachinski V, Lassen MA, Marshall J. Multi-infarct dementia. Lancet 1974; 2:207-210.

Hollister LE, Yesavage J. Ergoloid mesylates for senile dementia. Ann Intern Med 1984;100:894-898.

Horowitz GR. What is a complete work-up for dementia? Clin Geriatr Med 1988;4:163-180.

McKhann G, Drachman D, Folstein M, Katzman R, Price D, Stadlan EM. Clinical diagnosis of Alzheimer's disease: report of the NINCDS-ADRDA work group under the auspices of the Department of Health and Human Services Task Force on Alzheimer's Disease. Neurology 1984;34:939-944.

Rosen WG, Terry RD, Fuld PA, et al. Pathological verification of eschemic score in differentiation of dementias. Ann Neurol 1980;7:486-488.

Shuttleworth EC. Atypical presentations of dementia of the Alzheimer type. J Am Geriatr Soc 1984;32:485-490.

The Hastings Center. Guidelines on the termination of life-sustaining treatment and the care of the dying. Briarcliff Manor, New York, 1987.

Vinters HV, Miller BL, Pardridge WM. Brain amyloid and Alzheimer disease. Ann Intern Med 1988;109:41-54.

Two Women with Advanced Dementia

Case 9.

A. A 77-year-old woman with a history of several strokes has lost the ability to swallow. She is bedridden, incontinent, and suffers from advanced multi-infarct dementia.

She worked for many years as a clerk in a hospital, and cared for two relatives while they died of cancer. On many occasions she expressed her feelings opposing artificial life support, saying that she did not ever want to be a burden to anyone and felt that being kept alive by machines was "monstrous." Her physician wants to insert a nasogastric tube, but her two daughters, both nurses, refuse, stating that doing so would be contrary to their mother's wishes.

B. An 84-year-old woman with hypertension, heart disease, diabetes, and peripheral vascular disease is living in a nursing home. She has necrotic ulcers and gangrenous areas of her left foot, leg, and hip. She suffers from progressive dementia and is now bedridden and incontinent, and has severe contractures. She is unable to swallow enough food and water to maintain herself, and a nasogastric tube is inserted.

The patient has never been married. Her only surviving blood relative is a nephew who had known her for 50 years, and who was appointed her legal guardian when she was deemed incompetent. He had refused to allow amputation 2 years before, stating that it would have been counter to her wishes, and the patient survived. Now he feels that the nasogastric tube is of little longterm avail, and he requests that it be removed and his aunt be allowed to die. He cites the fact that she has always mistrusted doctors, and in the past, had expressed the desire to die in her own home.

of progressive but incomplete loss of cerebral cortical function. However, severely demented patients experience a truly vegetative existence that is often difficult to distinguish from PVS. In at least one jurisdiction, patients with PVS and those with dementia are governed by different legal standards, despite the fact that the difference is not always so vast from a neurological point of view that clinical decisions must arbitrarily rest on these differences.

4. An advance directive such as a "Living Will," "proxy designation," or "durable power of attorney for medical treatment," executed while the individual is competent, provides written proof of a patient's wishes regarding medical treatment, if the time comes that the patient lacks the capacity to make these decisions. A Living Will delineates these wishes, while a durable power of attorney or proxy designation appoints a trusted individual who should make health care decisions. As a practical matter, advance directives are more likely to be heeded if a state law exists. In states such as New York and New Jersey, which have a body of "case law" governing the right to refuse treatment, but lack a state statute, these documents would be highly reliable evidence of a patient's wishes. The O'Connor decision indicated that a Living Will would have been an ideal way for the patient to have expressed her wishes, since a written document shows that the person took the decision seriously. Unfortunately, there are thousands of patients with dementia who do not have written documents, even in states with statutes, and it would be unrealistic to demand documentation.

Pearls:

1. As of June 1989, 41 states and the District of Columbia have enacted legislation offering guidelines on when treatment can be stopped. Some states have both a "Living Will law" and a "health care agency (proxy) act," while one (Rhode Island) has only the latter. While a Living Will can stand on its own as instructions on life-sustaining treatment, a proxy designates a person to make these decisions. In New Jersey and New York, which currently lack such legislation, abundant court decisions ("case law") have made advance directives in effect, binding. In a few states with neither legislation nor local court decisions, the case law of other states is expected to act as "persuasive authority," granting advance directives a reality. The advantage of a statute is not only that it ensures a patient's right to refuse treatment, but it also protects the physician and the institution from liability if they comply with a patient's wishes. The latter is very important in the litigious atmosphere in which medicine is practiced today, since fear of liability often impels health providers to impose treatment that they and their patients may consider inappropriate.

Clue:

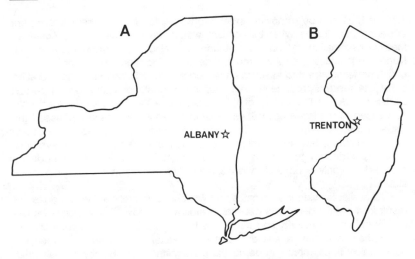

Questions:

1. Is it legal or ethical for the physician or nurse to withhold or withdraw nasogastric feeding in either case? Why or why not?

2. Do cases A and B differ from one another? Explain.

3. How are these patients similar or different from patients in a persistent vegetative state (PVS)?

4. Would the presence of an advance directive, such as a "Living Will," change matters?

Answers:

1. The tube can be removed under a physician's orders if there is sufficient evidence that this is what the patient would have wanted. The American Medical Association, the American Academy of Neurology (AAN), the American Nurses' Association, the Alzheimer's Disease Association, and other groups of health professionals and ethicists have held that artificial nutrition and hydration constitute medical treatments that may be withheld or withdrawn in certain situations. As of the writing of this book, the AAN statement is specifically addressed to the issue of PVS, while other organizations have addressed the issue in a more general way. This stance is generally reflected in the courts and legislatures, but not unanimously, presumably because of the symbolic meaning attributed to food and water. In addition, the level of evidence required to verify a patient's wishes may vary among the courts in various states.

All available evidence indicates that withdrawal of artificial feeding does not result in a painful death. In debilitated elderly, moreover, dehydration rapidly results in hyperosmolarity and coma, the former because of impaired ability of the kidney to conserve salt and water, the latter due to severe underlying neurological impairment. In dementia, nasogastric feeding may be painful or frightening, and patients often require restraints to prevent them from pulling out the tube. Patients in PVS, on the other hand, are incapable of experiencing pain, fear, and suffering, since destruction of the cerebral cortex is complete.

The stance of professional organizations and the courts notwithstanding, individual patients and health professionals have personal views regarding the still controversial issue of artificial feeding in dementia. Thus, there is no answer to question 1 that will satisfy everyone.

2. The patients in these two cases both have advanced dementia, although patient B may have a poorer medical prognosis than patient A. In both cases, there was disagreement between parties that could only be resolved in court. In both cases, the family members felt that artificial feeding would be opposed to the patient's wishes, while the health providers felt the procedure was required. Both eventually became landmark cases.

Case B is the famed "Claire Conroy case," which reached the New Jersey Supreme Court, and was one of the first cases in which it was ruled that there is no difference between artificial feeding and other forms of life support. This was also the first "right-to-die" case involving an adult who lacked decisional capacity because of dementia. Previous landmark cases dealt with patients who could not make medical decisions because of PVS, mental retardation, or other impairments. This case also reaffirmed the notion that there is no legal distinction between withholding or withdrawing treatment. Subsequent court

cases have generally reaffirmed this stance, and extended these prote patients whose lifespan was uncertain.

Case A took place in a different state (New York), and was decide differently. This was the case of Mary O'Connor, in which the state's court reversed two lower court decisions, and mandated that a tu inserted. The Decision held that there was not "clear and convincing ev from her numerous statements regarding abhorrence of artificial life supp she was opposed to artificial feeding in advanced dementia. The Court rule on the basis of prognosis, but on evidence of the patient's prev articulated wishes, which her family members were not allowed to inte The "clear and convincing" standard of New York state is more rigid tha standard of "substituted judgment" applied in other states, such as New Je in which a spokesperson is able to assert, in his or her best judgment, an incompetent patient would have wanted. Thus, cases that were clin similar, with evidence as to the patient's wishes comparable (perhaps weaker in case B than in case A), were decided quite differently in court law. The courts were acting to protect patient autonomy, and med decisions were secondary.

Occasionally, the "best interests" standard is applied in court, as in Arizona case, in which no one knew the patient, an elderly woman with multi neurological impairments, but tube feeding was stopped because it was fou to be consistent with her best interests.

The importance given to artificial feeding varies among the various sta legislatures as well. Several Living Will statutes (e.g., Colorado, Georgi Missouri, and Wisconsin) specifically exclude artificial feeding and hydratic from procedures that may be withheld or withdrawn based on a writte directive, namely, a Living Will. Regardless of the precise wording of Livin Will statutes, appellate courts have virtually unanimously upheld the patient's right to reject artificial feeding, as any other treatment, when there is evidence of the patient's wishes (but see Pitfall 2, below). Some of these cases were decided in states with apparently restrictive statutes, but the courts ruled that individuals still have rights (such as the constitutional right of self-determination) that would permit the withholding or withdrawal of feeding regardless of the statute.

3. PVS is a state of permanent eyes-open unconsciousness that results from complete and irreversible damage to the cerebral cortex. Brainstem functions such as respiration, pupillary responses, maintenance of circulation, and, sometimes, swallowing are maintained, and patients have been known to survive in this state for prolonged periods of time, the longest duration reported being 37 years. Patients with far-advanced dementia (sometimes called "end-stage dementia") can be neurologically very similar. One neurologist describes PVS as "amentia," to distinguish it from the "dementia" that occurs as a result

2. Although Claire Conroy died while the case was pending (the petition, granted by the trial court, had been denied by the Appellate Court), the New Jersey Supreme Court decided that it was important to rule in this case because it would have a bearing on many patients in the future. Death of the patient during litigation has been a common occurrence in landmark "right-to-die" cases.   Mary O'Connor is still alive, at the writing of this book.   Her nasogastric tube has fallen out many times, and her hands are restrained.

3. Nasogastric tubes should not be inserted in dementia patients with deglutition disorders for the sole indication of preventing aspiration pneumonia. The nasogastric tube worsens, rather than improves deglutition. Regurgitated food, saliva, and oropharyngeal bacteria will be aspirated more easily under these conditions.

Pitfalls:

1. Whenever involved parties disagree, even the directives of a Living Will or patient surrogate may not suffice, and if the case cannot be resolved by institutional conflict mediation, it must be resolved in court. This holds true whether or not the patient resides in a state that has enacted Living Will legislation.   Going to court is a method that is obviously cumbersome, time-consuming, and often prohibitively expensive, and is repeatedly discouraged by the courts themselves. As physicians and health care administrators become more informed of legal duties and protections, more cases will be resolved at the bedside, as they were before the advent of technology that required such decisions.

2. In January 1989, the Supreme Court of the State of Missouri ruled that Nancy Cruzan, a young woman in PVS for 5 years, could not have her feeding tube removed because the state's interest in the "preservation of life" was more important than the constitutional right of self-determination. Although the patient did not have a Living Will, the decision reflected the spirit of Missouri's Living Will statute, which considers artificial feeding to be ordinary care rather than medical treatment. This is the first high court case to rule in this way, and is considered problematic by physicians, since a medical decision was made on a narrow legal point, by a court, rather than between physician and the patient's family. The ruling is, furthermore, in conflict with official positions of established medical organizations.

3. Disagreement on termination of treatment is sometimes due to lack of communication rather than difference in philosophy.   Patients or their spokespersons may misunderstand the medical situation, and may change their position when the medical facts are clarified. The physician or the hospital may

misunderstand the law, which, if clarified, may dispel fear of liability. Because of jurisdictional differences and the developing nature of the law, it is useful for uncertain practitioners to "get a second opinion." For example, a physician may refuse to honor a Living Will because "it isn't legal in this state," while the absence of an actual statute does not mean that the document has no meaning.

4. Decisions not to resuscitate an incompetent, hopelessly ill patient in the event of cardiac or pulmonary arrest require consultation with close family members or other spokesperson, and not the more rigid evidence sometimes required in other termination-of-treatment questions. The Joint Commission of Accreditation of Healthcare Organizations has laid out specific guidelines for "DNR," and one state (New York) even has a law. Many physicians are opposed to DNR policies and laws because of the fear that rigid guidelines and demands for more paperwork will result in inappropriate resuscitations, a concern that merits study.

5. Percutaneous endoscopic gastrostomy (PEG) is an invasive but relatively well-tolerated method that is increasingly used to place feeding tubes in dementia patients. Although a gastrostomy tube is more comfortable for the patient than a nasogastric tube, restraints may still be required. Moreover, gastrostomy feeding does not appear to reduce risk of aspiration, because the patient does not control the amount of food being instilled, and because patients with deglutition disorders and impaired cough reflex remain unable to swallow or clear oropharyngeal secretions.   Finally, the decision of whether to feed by gastrostomy hinges on the same ethical and legal considerations as does the use of nasogastric feeding--namely, whether the decision to perform the procedure is in accordance with the patient's wishes, and whether the benefits of the treatment outweigh its burdens.

6. PVS and other states of permanent unconsciousness must be distinguished from "brain death," in which brainstem functions are also lost. When whole brain death occurs, an individual is considered legally dead.

References:

Alzheimer's Disease and Related Disorders Association, Inc. ADRDA policy statement on the treatment of patients with advanced dementia, 1985.

American Academy of Neurology, Position of the American Academy of Neurology on certain aspects of the care and management of the persistent vegetative state patient, April, 1988.

American Medical Association, Council on Ethical and Judicial Affairs, March 15, 1986.

Arras JD. The severely demented, minimally functional patient: an ethical analysis. J Am Geriatr Soc 1988; 36:938-944.

Billings JB. Comfort measures for the terminally ill: is dehydration painful? J Am Geriatr Soc 1985;33:808-810.

Ciocon JO, Silverstone FA, Graver M, Foley CJ.   Tube feeding in elderly patients.   Indications, benefits, and complications.   Arch Intern Med 1988;148:429-433.

Cranford RE. Termination of treatment in the persistent vegetative state. Semin Neurol 1984;4:36-44.

Epstein M, Hollenberg NK. Age as a determinant of renal sodium conservation in normal man. J Lab Clin Med 1976;87:411-417.

In re Conroy, 98 N.J. 321, 486 A.2d 1209 (1985).

Joint Commission on Accreditation of Healthcare Organizations, Withholding of resuscitative services, in Accreditation Manual 1989:82.

Lazaroff AE, Orr WF. Living wills and other advance directives. Clin Geriatr Med 1986;2:521-534.

Matter of O'Connor, 72 NY 2d 517 (1988).

Plum F, Posner JB. The diagnosis of stupor and coma. Philadelphia: FA Davis, 1980:1-16.

President's Commission for the study of ethical problems in medicine and biomedical and behavioral research, Deciding to forego life-sustaining treatment, 1983:190.

Rowe JW. Aging and renal function. In: Arieff AI, DeFronzo R. Fluid electrolyte and acid-base disorders. New York: Churchill Livingstone, 1985:969-1040.

Rowe JW, Shock NW, DeFronzo RA. The influence of age on the renal response to water deprivation in man. Nephron 1976;17:270-278.

Society for the Right to Die. The physician and the hopelessly ill patient: legal, medical, and ethical guidelines. New York, 1985; 1988 Supplement.

Steinbrook R, Lo, B. Artificial feeding--solid ground, not a slippery slope. N Engl J Med 1988;318:286-290.

Pseudodementia

Case 10.   A 79-year-old woman presents with urosepsis and diabetic hyperosmolar coma, She is adequately treated, but, after recovering, is thought by her physicians to have dementia.   A son, who lives in a town 200 miles away, reports that his mother had a 20-year history of type II diabetes, but stopped taking her tolbutamide "long ago" because she felt she didn't need it. She had always been "difficult," he says, tending to depression.   He is not surprised by the diagnosis of dementia.

Resumption of tolbutamide in the hospital is ineffective, but glucose is well controlled on daily NPH insulin, 20 units.   The patient is sent home where care is provided by her frail, 85-year-old husband and an experienced 12-hour home attendant who has had 1 year of nurse's training.   The home attendant volunteers to administer insulin and do blood glucose monitoring as well.

At home, the patient is said to be restless, claims that she is "always hungry," and is even up at night raiding the refrigerator.   She is forgetful, requires assistance with virtually all activities of daily living, and spends her day in aimless behavior, complaining, and, according to the husband, "driving everybody nuts."   Blood sugars performed at home by finger stick are almost always around 140 to 180 mg/dL.

The patient is slender and appears restless but alert.   Her blood pressure is 120/80, pulse is 70 and regular.   Neurologic examination is normal.   She is not terribly cooperative and seems disoriented but, on questioning, she remembers the date, day of the week, and year; knows her address; and knows the name of the hospital.   She addresses her new doctor by name (a foreign-sounding, multisyllable name) several times during the interview, without prompting.   When asked the name of the president, she wails, "Oh, I don't know!" and then whimpers, "Why can't I go home?"

On the basis of mental status testing, the diagnosis of dementia is questioned.   Amitriptyline, 12.5 mg at bedtime, is begun.   After 2 weeks, the home attendant reports that there may be some improvement and the dose is increased to 25 mg.   One week later, the patient reportedly is extremely weak and can't get out of bed.

53

Clue:

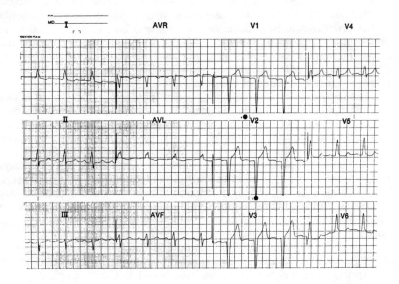

Questions:

1. What factors have led to the decision to treat with a tricyclic antidepressant (TCA)?

2. What are the dangers of this decision for this patient?

3. What are the alternatives to TCAs?

4. What are the alternatives to insulin?

Answers:

1. The treating physician feels that the patient is suffering from depression rather than dementia. Factors leading to this diagnosis are the lifelong "tendency to depression," the patient's better-than-expected performance on the mental status examination, and her dysphoria. Although the patient "acts" demented, her memory problem may well be secondary to the affective disorder. In dementia, memory loss is the primary problem and may result in secondary problems, such as depression or paranoia.

2. TCAs slow cardiac conduction through the electrical system. This effect is greatest in the His-Purkinje tissue and complete heart block can result. The patient's obvious conduction disease (right bundle branch block, left axis deviation, borderline first degree block) was present before the TCA was instituted and prompted the physician to initiate a subtherapeutic dose, but inpatient monitoring might have been a sensible measure. The drug was stopped in this patient 1 week after the dose was increased because the side effects that did develop (oversedation and orthostatic hypotension) were intolerable, as they often are in elderly patients. Amitriptyline was selected because of its sedative effect. Desipramine or nortriptyline 10 mg might have been a better choice because they have a lower tendency to cause orthostatic hypotension. Although they are less sedating, this characteristic is desirable when treating patients with apparent memory loss. However, if she had tolerated higher doses, a serious conduction problem might have developed. Perhaps her early side effects also protected her from anticholinergic problems that develop in elderly patients when they take anticholinergic TCAs such as amitriptyline, doxepin, and imipramine.

3. Monoamine oxidase inhibitors (MAOIs) are highly effective in elderly patients with depression and, because they do not slow cardiac conduction, may be used in patients with conduction disease. The most feared adverse effect-- hypertensive crisis related to tyramine or drug-drug interactions--occurs rarely, but would be an important consideration in this noncompliant patient, who should receive such medication only in a protected environment. MAOIs are less likely than TCAs to cause orthostatic hypotension, but far more likely to cause supine hypotension. The patient has a low-normal blood pressure for an elderly person, giving little margin for error. Alprazolam, a benzodiazepine with antidepressant activity, is sometimes useful, but unfortunately, is not as effective for major depressive disorders as the other agents.

Electroconvulsive therapy (ECT) is well tolerated in geriatric patients with depression and is often effective in major depression. Unfortunately, the required muscle-paralyzing agent succinylcholine could precipitate heart block in this patient, and a pacemaker might be required. ECT may be given in patients with pacemakers if close cardiologic supervision is obtained; premedication may need to be modified and strict attention to electrical circuitry is required. Psychotherapy is useful in some elderly patients with depression, but its relative efficacy compared to pharmacologic treatment and ECT in major depression has not been well studied.

4. Although the patient has type II diabetes, she is one of many patients who "escape" from the hypoglycemic effect of sulfonylurea agents over time, becoming insulin dependent. The reason that oral agents lose their efficacy in so many patients is not known. Although the "second generation" agents, glyburide and glipizide, are more potent on a milligram per milligram basis than the older agents, they cannot be relied upon to salvage treatment failures, which are usually due to weight gain, stress, underlying illness, or "escape." Occasional patients who fail to respond to one sulfonylurea do respond to another, however. There was no evidence that this patient's "hunger" was related to hypoglycemia and nocturnal eating was probably related to her insomnia and psychological impairment. Withdrawal from insulin produced hyperglycemia, which was not controlled with other oral agents. Because she is not obese, weight loss is not indicated, and even if her behavior and environment produce adequate dietary control, she will probably require insulin.

Pearls:

1. Depression in the elderly often can present with cognitive deficits such as inattention, memory impairment, and slowness of mental processing. In its severe form, this syndrome may be difficult to distinguish from dementia and has been termed "pseudodementia." The concept has not been well defined and is controversial because depression and dementia commonly coexist in the elderly. The important thing to remember is that this dementia-like illness is potentially reversible if the depression is adequately treated.

2. Except for the mental status examination, the neurologic examination may be otherwise normal in dementia and depression. The mental status test, a history suggestive of good cognitive function until recently, and the clinician's observations are probably the most reliable means of distinguishing between dementia and pseudodementia due to depression. The patient with Alzheimer's dementia generally is not dysphoric unless secondary depression exists and often cleverly deflects questions ("Oh, my husband can answer that") or answers incorrectly ("Franklin Roosevelt!"). A depressed patient often will not answer at all, or, looking dejected, might say, "I just don't know." On formal mental status tests, the demented patient tends to score lowest, the depressed patient scores highest, and the depressed patient with cognitive impairment

usually has an intermediate score. These tendencies reflect average scores, however, and are not accurate predictors of underlying pathology.

Another important clue to the diagnosis in these cases is that patients with AD usually do not complain of memory loss, while patients with depression generally are aware of a memory deficit and it can be the chief complaint. In elderly patients, the diagnosis may be confounded by the fact that dementia and depression not uncommonly coexist.

3.   Monoamine oxidase activity in the brain increases with age, lending theoretical support for the use of MAOIs in geriatric depression.

Pitfalls:

1.   TCAs are often inappropriately withheld from patients under the general category of "heart disease." Certainly they must be used with extreme caution, if at all, in patients with disease of the His-Purkinje system; patients with coronary insufficiency or uncompensated congestive heart failure could deteriorate if orthostatic hypotension were to develop. Even the young and physically healthy can develop serious cardiac complications from overdose. At therapeutic doses, they have a quinidine-like effect and reduce ectopy rather than produce it, do not depress the myocardium, and can be used safely in many patients if care is exercised. Initial dose should be very low and increases made slowly.

2.   Although sedating TCAs may relieve the insomnia that often complicates depression, they are not indicated as hypnotics in nondepressed patients. The TCAs are structurally related to the phenothiazines and confer sedation that is qualitatively similar. This, coupled with their long duration of action, may lead to an unpleasant "hangover" in the nondepressed insomniac.

3.   Medical treatment of depressed patients who "act demented" is complicated by the fact that TCAs can worsen confusion in some patients. Cognitive decline in Alzheimer's disease is thought to be related to central cholinergic deficits. TCAs rapidly enter the brain where their central anticholinergic effect can worsen or even precipitate dementia. TCA-induced dementia is reversible.

4.   In many localities, home attendants and home health aides are poorly paid, unskilled workers, and even the "best and the brightest" are not permitted by their vending agencies to administer medication of any type, presumably because of fear of legal liability. Nursing agencies are willing to train family members, but elderly spouses are often debilitated themselves and children all too often live far away. Dependent elderly patients, who are not lucky enough to employ an altruistic home attendant willing to administer medication "under

the table" (the present patient was one of the lucky ones) usually receive adequate care only after a medical disaster occurs and they end up in the hospital. Geriatricians generally favor the development of a professional corps of home health workers as a partial solution to this problem.

References:

Bidder TG. Electroconvulsive therapy in the medically ill patient. Psychiatr Clin North Am 1981;4:391-405.

Gerich JE. Sulfonylureas in the treatment of diabetes mellitus--1985. Mayo Clin Proc 1985;60:439-443.

Goldman LS, Alexander RC, Luchins DJ. Monoamine oxidase inhibitors and tricyclic antidepressants: comparison of their cardiovascular effects. J Clin Psychiatr 1986;47:225-229.

Karlinsky H, Shulman KI. The clinical use of electroconvulsive therapy in old age. J Am Geriatr Soc 1984;32:183-186.

Robinson DS, Davis JM, Nies A, Ravaris CL, Sylwester D. Relation of sex and aging to monoamine oxidase activity of human brain, plasma, and platelets. Arch Gen Psychiatr 1971;24:536-539.

Ruegg RG, Zisook S, Swerdlow NR. Depression in the aged: an overview. Psychiatr Clin North Am 1988;11:83-99.

Failure to Thrive

<u>Case 11.</u>   An 82-year-old woman is brought to your tertiary care hospital clinic by her daughter. The patient has had anorexia, weakness, weight loss, and fluctuating mental status for 9 months, and during this time has been hospitalized three times for episodes of depressed consciousness and urinary and fecal incontinence. During the hospitalizations she was afebrile and had normal blood count, chemistries, and CT scan of the brain. She has not had a cough, fever, sweats, or tachycardia.

Physical examination reveals a nonobese elderly woman who appears depressed and disoriented. Her complexion is sallow. Temperature is 99°F. Blood pressure and pulse are normal. She has kyphosis and a grade II/VI holosystolic murmur heard best at the apex and the left sternal border. Her lungs are clear. Her abdomen is slightly protuberant but nontender.

Laboratory evaluation reveals a hemoglobin of 11.9%, white blood count of 8000 cells/mm³, BUN of 35 mg/dL, creatinine of 1.4 mg/dL, and serum albumin of 2.7 g/dL. Erythrocyte sedimentation rate (ESR) is 40 mm/hr. Urinalysis is normal except for moderate proteinuria.

<u>Clue:</u>

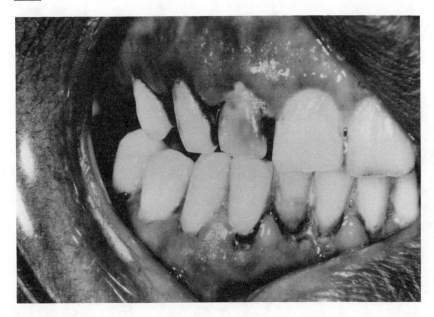

Questions:

1. What are the causes of "failure to thrive" in the elderly?

2. What aspects of the physical examination are particularly important in this patient?

3. What are the causes of mitral regurgitant murmurs in the elderly?

Answers:

1. "Failure to thrive," a nonspecific presentation characterized by weight loss, weakness, or other symptoms of inanition that do not point to a specific organ system, may be caused by many diseases in the elderly. Cancer, depression, hyperthyroidism, and tuberculosis are the diseases most often implicated. This patient was found to have streptococcus viridans (S. viridans) endocarditis, the subtle presentation diverting her diagnosticians from the actual disease. Treatment with penicillin reversed all of her symptoms as well as her mild laboratory abnormalities and she was able to return to her home where she resided on her own.

2. A careful search should be made for the source of the infection. Sites of infection in the elderly that are commonly overlooked include the mouth, the toes, the skin, the abdomen, and the pelvis. Dental caries in the elderly may be far advanced before pain occurs, and often form on the root surface. Skin ulcers, cellulitis, osteomyelitis, smouldering gallbladder disease, endometritis, or other pelvic disease may all lead to bacteremia and endocarditis. No source is "found" in over 50%, as in younger age groups.

3. Mitral incompetence in the elderly may still be rheumatic in origin, but nowadays is more often due to ischemic papillary muscle dysfunction. Other causes of mitral regurgitant murmurs are calcified mitral annulus (which may occur without demonstrable regurgitation) and typical mitral valve prolapse.

Pearls:

1. Although pre-existing valve disease can be identified in the majority of elderly patients with endocarditis, no underlying pathology can be found in up to 40% at autopsy.

2. Although gingival and dental infections can be due to a number of different organisms, including gram negative bacilli and anaerobes, S. viridans is the one typically implicated in oropharyngeal-associated endocarditis.

3. It is not uncommon for endocarditis and other infections to present without fever in the elderly (see Case 13).

4. Antibiotic prophylaxis is recommended in patients with heart murmurs, who are about to undergo dental procedures in which hematogenous seeding of bacteria may occur. However, it is not often appreciated that bacteremia may occur in ordinary gum chewing and toothbrushing, with nearly the frequency that it occurs during dental procedures. Prophylaxis, of course, was not at

issue with this patient, whose endocarditis was related to inadequate dental care, an extremely common problem among the elderly. The present case illustrates and underscores the need of elderly patients to have regular dental care.

5. The incidence of root (cervical) caries increases markedly with age. Root caries are distinguished from coronal caries by their location, and often go unnoticed unless a specific examination is made of this location. Gingival recession exposes the root surface of teeth to the oral environment, making the surface susceptible to destructive lesions. Dental care in the United States has improved to the extent that increasing numbers of older adults retain their teeth. Along with this dental longevity has come an increase in the prevalence of gingival recession. Age and gingival recession are the major risk factors in the development of root caries. It is not yet known whether dietary factors or age-related factors, such as changes in oral microbial flora, are important in their development.

Pitfalls:

1. As mentioned elsewhere in this book, thoracic deformities such as kyphosis can confuse the interpretation of heart murmurs in the elderly, so that aortic murmurs are often heard in the mitral area. However, this mitral murmur was, in fact, a mitral murmur.

2. The extremely high prevalence of systolic murmurs in the elderly (possibly 80% in those 80 years of age and older) should not divert attention from the significance of a murmur in a patient with cardiac or subtle systemic symptoms.

3. In addition to "typical" presentations, such as congestive heart failure, presentations of bacterial endocarditis in the elderly may include alteration in mental status, weight loss, anorexia, myalgias, uremia, and fever of unknown origin. Septic cerebral emboli in the elderly are sometimes misdiagnosed as typical atheroembolic strokes. Although these presentations may occur in younger adults, nonspecific symptoms lead to diagnostic difficulty because of their subtlety as well as their resemblance to other common diseases of late life.

References:

Applefield MM, Hornick RB. Infective endocarditis in patients over age 60. Am Heart J 1974;88:90-94.

Berman P, Fox RA. Fever in the eldery. Age Ageing 1985;14:327-332.

Cantrell M, Yoshikawa TT. Aging and infective endocarditis. J Amer Geriatr Soc 1983;31:216-222.

Everett ED, Hirschmann JV. Transient bacteremia and endocarditis prophylaxis. A review. Medicine 1977;56:61-77.

Kolibash AJ, Bush CA, Fontana MB, Ryan JM, Kilman J, Wooley CF. Mitral valve prolapse syndrome: analysis of 62 patients aged 60 or over. Am J Cardiol 1983;52:534-539.

Prutt AA, Rubin RH, Karchmer AW, Duncan GW. Neurologic complications of bacterial endocarditis. Medicine 1978;57:329-343.

Seichter U. Root surface caries: a critical literature review. J Amer Dent Assoc 1987;115:305-310.

Thell R, Martin FH, Edwards JE. Bacterial endocarditis in subjects 60 years of age and older. Circulation 1975;51:174-182.

Cachexia

Case 12. An 80-year-old man visits his doctor complaining that he has been constipated for a week. When he moved his bowels there was blood on the toilet tissue but he had no other gastrointestinal symptoms or prior history of severe constipation. He admits to anorexia for several weeks, has been unable to sleep, and thinks he has lost "a lot of weight." The patient has a history of systolic heart murmur and colonic polyps, and was recently diagnosed as having systolic hypertension for which hydrochlorothiazide was prescribed.

He has no history of surgery, psychiatric illness, blood transfusions, or drug or alcohol abuse. He denies fevers, palpitations, and cough, but has recently had two episodes of substernal pain radiating to the left arm, which he feels were brought on by anxiety. Electrocardiogram during these episodes revealed left ventricular hypertrophy by voltage criteria, and was unchanged from previous EKGs.

On physical examination, the patient has kyphosis and is cachectic. Blood pressure is 120/80. Pulse is 88 and regular. His thyroid gland is not palpable. There is no proptosis. Lungs are clear. There is a grade II/VI systolic ejection murmur heard at the base, without radiation. Abdomen is scaphoid; no masses are felt. Rectal examination is normal, and stool is guaiac negative. The patient weighs 120 pounds, 14 pounds less than 3 months before.

Blood tests are sent and a barium enema is scheduled.

Clue:

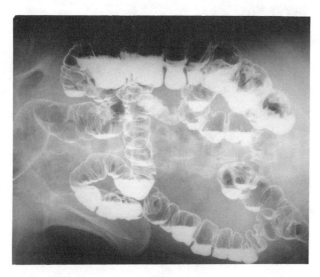

Questions:

1. What does this presentation look exactly like?

2. If it isn't that, what is it?

3. Why was the patient constipated?

4. What are the explanations for the heart murmur?

5. What medication is indicated prior to definitive treatment?

Answers:

1. This patient's marked weight loss and severe constipation suggest colon cancer, particularly in view of his history of colonic polyps. To his physician's surprise, the barium enema was normal.

2. The patient had thyrotoxicosis. An alert geriatric fellow ordered thyroid function tests, which revealed a T_4 of 19.1 μg/dL (N = 6.2-13.2), T3RU of 33% (N = 20-32), and TSH of 0.4 mIU/mL (N = 0.8-4.8). Radioactive iodine uptake was "low normal," but the scan revealed two demarcated areas in the left lobe intensely concentrating the radiopharmaceutical and suppressing the right lobe, and was considered diagnostic of hyperfunctioning nodules.

3. Although diuretic therapy might have been a contributing factor, the constipation was due to hyperthyroidism, and it resolved when the hyperthyroidism was treated. More than 20% of elderly hyperthyroid patients present with constipation, rather than classic symptoms of diarrhea or hyperdefecation. The mechanism is not known, but may be related to the increased number of beta adrenergic receptors that accompany hyperthyroidism. The increased beta sensitivity of gut smooth muscle would result in relaxation and inhibition of motility and perhaps constipation if the gut were predisposed. The tendency to develop constipation is common in healthy elderly probably explains part of this phenomenon.

4. Hyperthyroidism can produce a flow murmur or accentuate an existing murmur, but this patient's heart murmur antedated the onset of hyperthyroidism by years. Approximately 80% of 80 year olds have systolic murmurs, and the vast majority of these murmurs are not clinically important. Aortic valve murmurs in the elderly are generally due to disordered flow across a sclerotic or calcific, but not stenotic, valve. If the patient's symptoms were to subside after antithyroid treatment, significant aortic stenosis would be unlikely.

5. Antithyroid agents such as propylthiouracil or methimazole should be given prior to radioactive iodine since a transient rise in thyroid hormone levels may occur shortly after radioactive iodine treatment and could be harmful to someone with underlying cardiac disease. Such pretreatment is standard in geriatric practice because of the high incidence of overt and subclinical cardiac disease. Propranolol should be given to relieve symptoms of sympathetic discharge until the patient is euthyroid. Interestingly, this patient's constipation was relieved shortly after propranolol was instituted.

Pearls:

1. As many as 40% of hyperthyroid patients over 60, and up to 70% of those over 75, do not have tachycardia. This may be because of underlying conduction system disease or concurrent use of negative inotropic medications.

2. Kyphosis due to osteoporosis is uncommon in elderly men, the male-to-female ratio for this condition being 8 to 1.

3. Hyperthyroidism can accelerate bone loss and it is tempting to think that it may have been a contributing factor in this patient.

4. The presentation of hyperthyroidism in the elderly is often "monosystemic." This may have to do with the fact that many elderly have subclinical disease in at least one organ system and the most vulnerable organ is "hit" first. The cardiovascular system is often involved, and the patient can present with atrial fibrillation or congestive heart failure alone. Roughly 15% of hyperthyroid patients over the age of 60 present with the triad of weight loss, anorexia, and constipation, the "gastrointestinal" presentation described in this case.

5. Propranolol inhibits peripheral conversion of T_4 to active T_3 and can lower serum T_3 by 15 to 20%. It is not known whether reduction in symptoms results from this effect, from beta-blockade, or both.

Pitfalls:

1. When hyperthyroidism presents in late life, it is usually not due to Grave's disease, and so classic signs of Grave's disease such as goiter and exophthalmos are uncommon. The most common cause of hyperthyroidism in the elderly is toxic multinodular goiter, or a toxic nodule, but since the thyroid itself may be atrophic, or may lie below the clavicles, physical examination of the thyroid is often misleading.

2. The presence of a tremor in an elderly person is a nonspecific sign, and any kind of tremor can be accentuated by hyperthyroidism. The careful observer can note, however, that uncomplicated "senile" essential tremor has a lower frequency and greater amplitude than hyperthyroid tremor. Parkinsonian tremor is likewise different in quality and occurs in conjunction with other physical signs.

3. Age-related skeletal deformities, such as kyphosis, can alter internal thoracic anatomy. These anatomic changes are usually not medically important, but can confound the physical evaluation. For example, aortic murmurs can be heard

in the mitral region, and vice versa, or the thyroid gland can drop below the clavicle and evade the examiner.

4.   Longterm use of antithyroid medication can cause more problems in the elderly than the young, so radioactive iodine is the preferred treatment for the elderly patient with toxic nodules or Grave's disease. The disadvantage of definitive treatment is that the patient may be lost to followup and secondary hypothyroidism may go undetected until serious problems develop.

References:

Bilezikian JP, Loeb JN. The influence of hyperthyroidism and hypothyroidism on alpha- and beta-adrenergic receptor systems and adrenergic responsiveness Endocr Rev 1983;4:378-388.

Cooper DS, Ridgway EC. Clinical management of patient with hyperthyroidism. Med Clin N Amer 1985;69:953-970.

Davis PJ, David FB. Hyperthyroidism in patients over the age of 60 years. Medicine 53:161-181, 1974.

Tibaldi JM, Barzel US, Albin J, Surks M. Thyrotoxicosis in the very old. Amer J Med 1986;81:619-622.

Wong M, Tei C, Shah PM. Degenerative calcific valvular disease and systolic murmurs in the elderly. J Amer Geriatr Soc 1983;31:156-163.

Diarrhea

<u>Case 13.</u> An 84-year-old woman has suffered a stroke and is residing in a nursing home. She develops diarrhea and you are called to evaluate her. You find that she was evaluated the previous evening by the on-call physician who found "nothing significant," and performed a complete blood count (CBC). There are no other cases of diarrhea on her floor. She has a "PRN" order for a stool softener, acetaminophen, and milk of magnesia, but has not been on antibiotics recently.

On physical examination, the patient is lying in bed and smiles to greet you. She is slightly lethargic, but when you ask her how she feels she says, "Oh, not so bad."

On physical examination she is afebrile, and has a dense right hemiparesis. Examination of her lungs reveals coarse crepitations at both bases. Abdominal examination reveals somewhat decreased bowel sounds and mild tenderness. Rectal examination reveals no masses. Stool is brown and guaiac positive. The remainder of the physical examination is normal. According to the chart, the lung findings have been present since her admission a year ago. White blood count (WBC) from the previous evening is 16,000 cells/mm^3, and hematocrit is 40%. You send another CBC to the laboratory and continue your rounds.

Question:

What is the differential diagnosis?

Answer:

Diarrhea in a nursing home patient may be infectious, due to either contaminated food or person-to-person contact. An underrecognized cause of infectious diarrhea is bacterial contamination of liquid diets, which occurs less often in commercial feeds than in "home brew" preparations, and develops readily if the feed is not adequately refrigerated or used quickly enough. Bed- and wheelchair-bound patients frequently suffer from constipation and fecal impaction; the latter sometimes presents with diarrhea as loose stool is expelled around the impaction. Conversely, overtreatment with laxatives could have produced diarrhea in this patient. However, the high WBC in the presence of occult blood should raise the suspicion of diverticulitis or ischemic colitis.

After 3 hours, the laboratory calls to report that the repeat WBC is 35,000.

Clue:

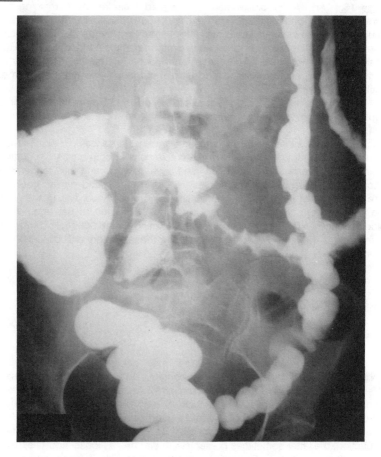

Questions:

1. What does the doubling of the white count prompt you to do?

2. Explain the patient's presentation.

Answers:

1. The marked increase in WBC in less than 24 hours requires an immediate reevaluation of the patient's status. On examination, she was still lethargic but not more than on the previous evaluation. Her abdomen was less soft and not markedly tender, but her bowel sounds were completely absent. An emergency surgical consultation was required because of the possibility of perforated viscus. Barium enema revealed "thumbprinting," a characteristic radiographic feature of acute colonic ischemia that represents submucosal hemorrhage and edema. Thumbprinting persists only until mucosal breakdown occurs, so that absence of thumbprinting does not rule out ischemic bowel. Conversely, persistence of thumbprinting beyond a few days suggests a different lesion.

At surgery, the patient underwent hemicolectomy for massive bowel infarction. Two days later she required repeat laparotomy for suspected repeat infarction, and died.

2. The patient's minimal symptoms in the face of an abdominal catastrophe is not unusual in elderly patients, particularly those who are neurologically impaired. Such subtle presentations are probably due to impaired perception or expression of pain, but they are by no means universal, since many elderly patients present in typical, textbook fashion.

Pearls:

1. The increased morbidity and mortality seen in elderly patients undergoing abdominal surgery is not due to age alone, but is due to underlying disease or surgical delay. Delay may be due to the subtle presentation of the pathology, fear of a negative outcome, and the desire to treat "expectantly," or because underlying disorders must be stabilized first. In the case of bowel infarction, however, overall mortality is 70%, even when surgery is prompt. Patients undergoing surgery still have at least a 50% mortality.

2. In addition to vascular occlusion, another important cause of ischemic bowel in the elderly is the "low flow" syndrome, in which congestive heart failure or hypotension impairs perfusion of the mesenteric bed. Hyperviscosity syndromes due to polycythemia vera or multiple myeloma are less common causes, but in all cases the elderly patient is expected to be at greater risk because of the high prevalence of underlying mesenteric artery stenosis in the geriatric population.

Pitfalls:

1. The absence or attenuation of fever in this and other infectious disease in the elderly is very common, and should not divert the diagnostician from considering infection. Alterations in immune response, decrease in the production of endogenous pyrogens, or abnormalities in thermoregulation have been proposed as causes of attenuated fever in the elderly. In addition, oral temperature measurement may be particularly unreliable in debilitated elderly because of the lack of cooperation or the presence of mouth breathing.

2. The presence of basilar crepitations in immobile elderly patients is common and can confuse the physical evaluation. Chronic crepitations are thought to be due to basilar alveolar atelectasis or scarring. If chronic, these findings need not cause alarm, but they may obscure new changes, such as the fine rales of pneumonia or heart failure.

References:

Berman P, Fox RA. Fever in the eldery. Age Ageing 1985;14:327-332.

Brandt LJ. Gastrointestinal disorders of the elderly. New York: Raven Press, 1984:396-421.

Charlesworth D. Surgery in old age. In: Brocklehurst JC, ed. Textbook of Geriatrics and Gerontology. 3rd ed. Edinburgh: Churchill Livingstone, 1985:935-957.

DeLeeuw IH, Vandewoude MF. Bacterial contamination of enteral diets. Gut 1986;27(S1):56-57.

Finucane PM, Arunachalam T, O'Dowd J, Pathy MSJ. Acute mesenteric infarction in elderly patients. J Amer Geriatr Soc 1989;37:355-358.

O'Connell TX, Kadell B, Tompkins RK. Ischemia of the colon. Surg Gyn Obstet 1976;142:337-342.

Hip Pain Six Months after Repair of a Hip Fracture

Case 14. A 79-year-old woman, born in Denmark, suffered from degenerative disc disease with chronic pain and difficulty ambulating. Three years ago she sustained a compression fracture of her L-1 vertebra when she slipped while trying to board a bus. Six months ago, she was standing uncomfortably for 20 minutes while waiting for a taxi when she developed severe pain in her right hip and fell to the ground. She was unable to bear weight on her affected leg and when she finally got a taxi, she took it directly to her doctor's office where an x-ray of the hip was done. The x-ray was said to be normal, but her symptoms persisted. Three days later she went to a local hospital emergency room where a repeat hip x-ray revealed a subcapital hip fracture. Hip surgery was performed 12 hours later and an Austin-Moore hemiprosthesis was inserted. Within a week she was able to ambulate with a walker, and within a few weeks, she was walking with a cane, although with somewhat more difficulty than before the hip fracture. Two weeks ago she began to notice pain in her right hip, and, disillusioned with her original physician because of the misdiagnosis, she comes to you for help. She has been well except for the fact that she underwent extraction of two "infected molars" one month ago.

On physical examination she is a slender Caucasian woman with normal blood pressure, pulse, and temperature. Her right leg is 1 inch shorter than her left. There is no erythema, swelling, or tenderness at the surgical site. She walks with a stooped posture and limps slightly "because of the pain."

She informs you that she underwent natural menopause at age 51, has a "hiatus hernia" for which she takes large doses of antacids, has mild hypertension for which she takes hydrochlorothiazide 50 mg per day, and has been treated for chronic idiopathic pruritus with ointments and intermittently with a "white pill." She proudly enumerates the array of vitamins and minerals that she takes daily, some in large doses, and it is obvious that she is well informed on the "latest" in nutritional therapy. She also takes 1500 mg of calcium carbonate per day on the advice of her orthopedic surgeon.

Clue:

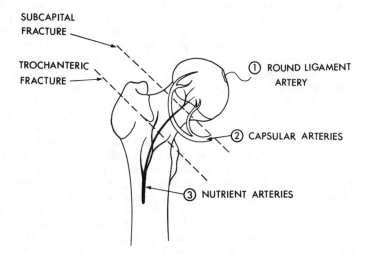

SUBCAPITAL
FRACTURE

TROCHANTERIC
FRACTURE

① ROUND LIGAMENT
ARTERY

② CAPSULAR ARTERIES

③ NUTRIENT ARTERIES

Questions:

1. What factors other than the patient's age and postmenopausal state could have contributed to her bone fragility?

2. When did the hip fracture occur?

3. Why was the first x-ray read as normal?

4. Why did her orthopedic surgeon insert an Austin-Moore hemiprosthesis and not perform the simpler repair with Knowles pins?

5. Why did he recommend such high doses of calcium?

6. What is the differential diagnosis of her <u>new</u> hip pain?

7. What medical treatment would you recommend for her bone disease?

Answers:

1. She is a Caucasian of northern European descent and at high risk for involutional osteoporosis, probably on a genetic basis. High doses of vitamin D may increase bone resorption. Hypervitaminosis A and high doses of fluoride may cause formation of abnormal, fragile bone. Aluminum-containing antacids (Mylanta, Riopan, Amphogel, others) cause phosphate depletion, which can impair mineralization of bone; prolonged ingestion of high doses may result in osteomalacia. Idiopathic pruritus is sometimes treated (inappropriately) with oral corticosteroids, which inhibit collagen synthesis and can result in osteoporosis. Slender stature and lack of physical exercise are independent risk factors for osteoporosis.

2. Hip fractures sometimes occur after apparently nontraumatic stress if the femoral neck is severely osteopenic. A patient may report struggling to break a fall and applying torsion to the hip, or may report no obvious trauma at all, so that the fall sometimes is caused by the fracture, and not the other way around. The patient in question probably fractured her hip while standing uncomfortably for a long time.

3. Not all fractures are immediately apparent on x-ray. Lateral and oblique views may be needed to confirm a fracture. Positional rotation may obscure radiographic signs of fractures. Early healing may make small fractures more apparent on x-ray several days later. Severe osteopenia and a "paper-thin" cortex are common radiographic features in the bones of elderly patients that make the classic x-ray findings of hip fracture less than obvious.

4. Subcapital fractures may cut off the major arterial blood supply to the femoral head since the artery of the round ligament provides adequate supply in only 5% of individuals (see Clue). Avascular necrosis of the femoral head occurs as a late complication in over 30% of subcapital fractures that have been nailed or pinned at surgery. Hemiprosthesis circumvents the problem of avascular necrosis because the femoral head is removed and replaced by the prosthesis. Moreover, the hemiprosthesis allows early weight bearing, speeding rehabilitation and lowering the likelihood of complications that occur as a result of prolonged bed rest.

5. Intestinal calcium absorption declines markedly with age, particularly in women. Between 1500 and 2000 mg of calcium are required to maintain positive calcium balance in old age. However, if this patient's average daily dietary intake had been considered in calculating the dose of calcium supplements, the dose might have been reduced. Whether or not calcium supplementation will reduce fracture risk at this age is a subject of debate.

6.   Loosening of the prosthesis in the femoral shaft may have occurred, or the prosthesis might have been the wrong "fit" for the patient's acetabulum.   Both factors could result in acetabular erosion and secondary osteoarthritis.   Latent infection around the prosthesis can present with pain in the absence of classic signs of infection.   Such infection can be introduced at the time of surgery or can be caused by bacteremia from a procedure such as a dental extraction. Hip x-rays, CBC with differential, and erythrocyte sedimentation rate should be done.   This patient was found to have early acetabular erosion on x-ray.

7.   Calcium should be continued if tolerated, because it is safe and will slow the rate of bone loss, although it is not as effective as estrogen in this regard. Estrogen will not reverse osteoporosis and, in general, is reserved for younger postmenopausal women in whom the beneficial effect on bone is well known. Fluoride has not been approved by the Food and Drug Administration for the treatment of osteoporosis and its use is currently under investigation.   Calcitonin has been approved, but it is expensive, must be given by injection, and has not yet been demonstrated to reduce the fracture rate in women with osteoporosis. Exercise should be encouraged as tolerated.   Modest sunlight exposure and physiologic (400-800 IU) doses of vitamin D should be given to ensure adequate intestinal calcium absorption.   Megavitamin A and D should be stopped.   Aluminum-containing antacids can be replaced by calcium carbonate antacids (Tums or Titralac), and the dose of other calcium supplements adjusted accordingly.   The "hiatal hernia" should be reevaluated.

Pearls:

1.   Avascular necrosis of the femoral head is almost unheard of in the setting of a trochanteric fracture since blood supply is not interrupted. These fractures are repaired by approximating the ends of the fracture with internal fixation.

2.   Lifelong high dietary intake of calcium probably retards bone loss, not simply by adding calcium to bone, but by promoting endogenous calcitonin secretion and reducing bone resorption.   Remember that bone consists of collagen as well as mineral.   In osteoporosis, collagen matrix and mineral are lost proportionately.

3.   Osteomalacia may be a component of bone disease in some elderly individuals, usually because of vitamin D deficiency. This is particularly common in countries where milk products are not fortified with vitamin D and where sunlight is low.   Osteomalacia is not caused by calcium lack.

4.   Thiazide diuretics may retard bone loss and decrease fracture rates by reducing renal calcium excretion.

5. A bone scan done 12 or more hours after hip trauma may reveal a subtle fracture not seen on plain x-ray.

Pitfalls:

1. Osteoporosis occurs later and to a much smaller degree in blacks than other races, but bone disease is common in Orientals and other nonblack races.

2. Osteophytes that form at the articular cartilage of the hip in patients with arthritis can have the radiographic appearance of a femoral neck fracture--a sclerotic line appearing to run across the femoral neck. Careful evaluation of medial and lateral femoral head-neck junction on the plain x-ray reveals smooth arcs in nonfractured hips. This smooth arc is usually disturbed or angulated when a fracture is present. Tomography can also help to distinguish an osteophyte from a fracture.

3. Although single- and dual-photon absorptiometry, and CT scanning of the spine are commonly used to determine bone mineral density in large studies, they are unreliable predictors of fracture risk in individual patients, and are currently not recommended for routine use in clinical practice. The presence or absence of certain risk factors for osteoporosis, such as age, race, body habitus, and family history, may be more reliable predictors than bone mineral determination.

References:

Attenborough CG. Fractures near the hip. In: Devas M, ed. Geriatric Orthopedics. London: Academic Press, 1977.

Bucholz RW. Injuries of the pelvis and hip. Emerg Med Clin North Am;1984;2:331-346.

Cummings SR, Black D. Should perimenopausal women be screened for osteoporosis? Ann Intern Med 1986;104:817-823.

Kavlie H, Sundal B. Primary arthroplasty in femoral neck fractures. Acta Orthop Scand 1974;45:579-590.

Riggs BL, Melton LJ. Involutional osteoporosis. N Engl J Med 1986;314:1676-1686.

Sisk TD.   Fractures of hip and pelvis. In: Crenshaw AH, ed. Campbell's operative orthopedics. CV Mosby, 1987:1719-1781.

Four Women in an Osteoporosis Clinic

Case 15.

A. A youthful 78-year-old Caucasian woman has kyphosis due to thoracic compression fractures. Her mother, who recently died at the age of 96, lived a healthy life, but, in the end, had profound osteoporosis and multiple fractures.

B. A 63-year-old nurse has suffered five compression fractures in the past few years. She is always in pain and takes the combination narcotic analgesic Percodan practically every day. She is obese, of European Jewish descent, and denies a family history of osteoporosis. She does not want to take estrogen because her sister died of endometrial carcinoma.

C. A 46-year-old slender Irish-American woman reports that her menstrual periods are "becoming erratic." She begins to think of impending menopause and wants to take estrogen to prevent osteoporosis, but she is afraid because her mother and maternal aunt had breast cancer.

D. A healthy 24-year-old Chinese-American medical student has been reading about osteoporosis and wants to know if she should be taking calcium supplements. Her fiance, who is a medical resident, told her she's "nuts," and that "Orientals don't get osteoporosis anyway."

Clue:

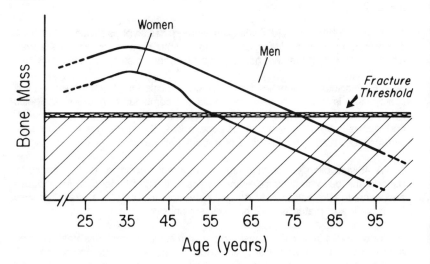

Questions:

1. What are the risk factors for progressive bone loss in each patient?

2. What would you advise them?

3. What are the side effects of treatment?

Answers:

A. This patient has established osteoporosis and her obvious risk factor is family history. If she lives as long as her mother did, her bones are likely to be as bad and preventive measures are indicated. A sensible program of exercise (preferably weight-bearing) should be prescribed. This patient, who already has spinal fractures, should walk regularly in rubber-soled shoes, which absorb impact.

Some bone loss can be prevented by increasing her calcium intake to 2000 mg of elemental calcium per day, including dietary intake. Intestinal calcium absorption declines with age and 1500 to 2000 mg are required to maintain zero calcium balance after the menopause in women. Calcium supplements are most efficiently given as calcium carbonate because this compound contains 40% elemental calcium and fewer tablets need to be taken to achieve the desired intake. Physiologic doses of vitamin D (400-800 IU daily) should be given to enhance intestinal calcium absorption, and to prevent osteomalacia, which may coexist with osteoporosis. Because of impaired calcium absorption, hypercalcemia and hypercalciuria are rare concomitants of calcium supplementation in elderly women. However, subclinical hyperparathyroidism is not rare, and anyone prescribed calcium supplements should have baseline and followup measurements of serum calcium.

Calcitonin increases bone mineral content and is assumed, but not proved, to reduce the fracture rate. Because of its safety, it can be recommended to this patient if she can afford it and doesn't mind injecting herself. The officially recommended dose is 100 IU daily subcutaneously, but a lower dose (50 IU 3 to 7 times a week) may be equally or more effective, is cheaper, is less likely to cause nausea, and improves compliance. Calcitonin's hypocalcemic effect may stimulate the parathyroid glands, so the regimen should include calcium supplements.

This is one of the few patients over 75 in whom estrogen might be considered. Estrogen does not rebuild osteopenic bone but retards postmenopausal bone loss. It has not been adequately studied in elderly women who have passed the "estrogen-sensitive" period of bone loss. The "estrogen-sensitive" period lasts roughly 7-8 years after menopause and is depicted in the Clue as a dip in the curve for women. Although some investigators feel that estrogen does not continue to forestall bone loss in late life, some evidence suggests that it may.

Fluoride is the only substance known to increase bone mass. However, it is not known if the new bone (fluoroapatite) is more or less fragile than untreated bone, and bone-building doses are very irritating to the gastrointestinal tract. The final word on fluoride awaits the outcome of prospective studies, and is not recommended at this time.

B. A patient without a family history of osteoporosis, and who, in addition, has the negative risk factor of obesity, requires a thorough workup and interview to uncover other processes that have produced her problem at a relatively young age. Workup failed to reveal other causes of osteopenia, such as multiple myeloma, hyperparathyroidism, hyperprolactinemia, or vitamin D-deficient osteomalacia. A drug history revealed that she had been taking high doses (5 grains per day!) of thyroid hormone from age 25 to age 50. This had been prescribed for presumed hypothyroidism. A more modern workup at age 50 revealed that her thyroid function was normal. Thyrotoxicosis enhances bone resorption and may result in osteoporosis. Thus, it is possible that high doses of thyroid hormone ("factitious hyperthyroidism") harmed this patient's bone.   Other causes of bone fragility include corticosteroids, heparin, and excessive doses of phosphate-depleting, aluminum-containing antacids or of vitamin A or D.

One cannot predict the patient's actual risk of developing endometrial carcinoma with estrogen therapy, but her fears regarding her risks should certainly be respected. Estrogen would not restore her osteopenic bone but would only prevent further deterioration. Even if she were highly motivated, she should not receive estrogen without first receiving an endometrial biopsy to rule out endometrial carcinoma or atypical hyperplasia. If she were to receive estrogen, it would have to be given in combination with progesterone, which reduces the risk of developing estrogen-induced endometrial pathology, and endometrial sampling would have to be done every 6 to 12 months. In addition to calcium, vitamin D, and exercise prescribed for patient A, this patient is a good candidate for calcitonin therapy since she has had experience administering injectable medication.   In addition, calcitonin may have a nonspecific effect on pain by increasing secretion of beta-endorphin.

C. This slender Caucasian woman is statistically at increased risk of developing osteoporosis and the early postmenopausal period is the ideal time to begin estrogen prophylaxis.   There is no evidence that estrogen therapy causes breast cancer de novo, but in view of her strong family history, it is probably prudent to avoid estrogen in this patient.

It is currently recommended that all women with intact uterus should receive progesterone along with estrogen, to prevent the development of endometrial cancer. The combination has no known cancer-causing or cancer-preventing effect on the breast.   Progesterones, however, can reverse the beneficial effect of estrogen on the lipid profile.   Estrogen increases high density lipoprotein cholesterol (HDLC) while synthetic progestogens currently in use decrease HDLC. Native progesterone does not have this adverse effect, but is poorly absorbed and is not yet available for general use.   As an alternative to estrogen, this patient should be counseled with regard to other controllable risk factors such as cigarette smoking, lack of exercise, low calcium diet, and bone-harming exogenous substances discussed above.

D.   This young woman is not "nuts," but she does not require calcium supplements unless her calcium intake is severely curtailed by conditions such as lactose intolerance or strong distaste for foods rich in calcium.   Her fiance is wrong, however, about the risk to Oriental women.   It is commonly assumed that the lighter one's complexion, the greater the risk for osteoporosis.   It is true that black men and women have a very low risk of osteoporosis, for reasons that are not understood but are presumably on a genetic basis. However, women of Chinese, Japanese, and related ancestry, have a significant risk.

The best advice for this woman is to increase her dietary calcium intake to at least 800 mg per day, the recommended daily allowance for young adults. Dietary calcium is reliably absorbed and is found not only in all milk products, but in green leafy vegetables and canned salmon and sardines. She should get as much physical exercise as possible, but should avoid extremes, since young marathon runners who exercise so much that they lose their menstrual periods may actually reduce bone mass.   She should also have adequate sunlight exposure.   No more than 15 minutes three times a week is required to maintain adequate vitamin D status, which is fortunate for sun-deprived people like medical students, interns, and homebound elderly.

References:

Eastell R, Riggs BL.   Treatment of osteoporosis. Obstet Gynecol Clin North Am 1987;14:77-88.

Drinkwater BN, Nilson KL, Chestnut CH.   Bone mineral content of amenorrheic and eumenorrheic athletes. N Engl J Med 1984;311:277-281.

Lindsay R.   Prevention of postmenopausal osteoporosis. Obstet Gynecol Clin North Am 1987;14:63-76.

McDermott MT, Kidd GS.   The role of calcitonin in the development and treatment of osteoporosis.   Endocr Rev 1987;8:377-390.

Riggs BL, Melton LJ.   Involutional osteoporosis.   N Engl J Med 1986;314:1676-1686.

Urinary Incontinence

<u>Case 16.</u>   An 84-year-old widow suffered a stroke, leaving her with flaccid left hemiplegia, and was transferred to a nursing home for rehabilitation. She had no aphasia and no apparent cognitive impairment but was very depressed. Her other medical problems included hypertension, severe osteoarthritis of the knees, urinary incontinence, and obesity.

Three months after the stroke her left arm and leg remained flaccid. She had urinary frequency but, except for occasional "leakage" when she was stood up, she remained continent if toileted regularly. Unfortunately, she could not bear adequate weight on her nonparalyzed leg because of troublesome pain and stiffness of the knee. This, plus her heavy weight, made it necessary for two people to toilet and transfer her. She was deeply embarrassed that her weight necessitated two-person assistance. This worsened her self-esteem and deepened her depression.

The patient came from a very close and loving family who visited her daily. Her daughter came by every day after work for 2 hours, and spent 4 to 5 hours on Saturday and Sunday. Elaborate plans were made so that the patient could live with the daughter and her family at home. The patient's son (who lived with his family in a city 400 miles away) declared his intention to look for work nearby so that he could assist in his mother's care. The actual care, it turned out, would be minimal, as long as the patient could be toileted.

Her medications included ibuprofen 600 mg q.i.d. for arthritis, prazosin 5 mg b.i.d. for hypertension, and desipramine 50 mg at bedtime for depression.

An incontinence plan was instituted in the nursing home and included medications, "bladder training," pelvic floor exercises, and incontinence garments. A 1000-calorie diet was abandoned when the patient repeatedly expressed anguish to staff and family that food was her "only pleasure," and her family brought her treats on a daily basis.

Clue:

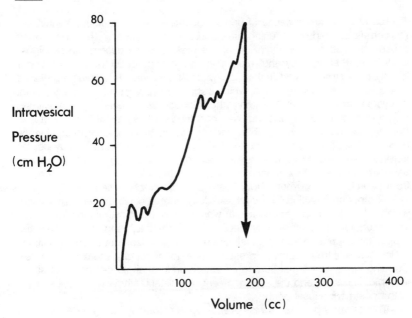

Questions:

1. What are the possible factors contributing to the patient's urinary dysfunction?

2. What nonpharmacologic approaches should be employed to keep this patient dry? What should be avoided?

3. What medications might alleviate her incontinence?

4. Could the patient be cared for at home? How?

Answers:

1. The most common cause of urinary incontinence in the elderly is unstable ("hyperreflexic," "spastic," "uninhibited neurogenic") bladder. This condition is caused by loss of tonic inhibition of the brainstem detrusor reflex by higher centers, so that urgency and micturition contractions occur when the bladder is only partially filled, earlier than in a normal bladder. This volume-pressure relationship is seen in the Clue, which depicts a hypothetical cystometrogram. A cystometrogram involves filling the bladder with water and measuring pressure as the bladder fills, but was not done on this patient because it was not felt that it would change her therapy. In unstable bladder, incontinence need not result, but dependent or physically disabled individuals may not be able to toilet themselves before expulsion of urine occurs. Unstable bladder usually develops in the absence of an obvious neurologic lesion, or may result from neurologic impairment, both being possible in this patient.

Another contributing factor in this elderly woman could be pelvic relaxation, which afflicts many postmenopausal women, producing "stress incontinence." The short female urethra may become "hypermobile," and drop below the urogenital diaphragm so that small amounts of urine leak out under conditions of increased intra-abdominal pressure due to a cough, sneeze, or merely standing up. The normal 90-degree vesico-urethral angle generally increases in pelvic relaxation, and the estrogen-sensitive distal urethra may also lose tone in the postmenopausal period.

This patient's physicians wisely refrained from treating her hypertension with diuretics, but failed to realize that prazosin may have contributed to her bladder problem. Internal urethral sphincter tone is enhanced by alpha-adrenergic stimulation. Alpha blockers, such as prazosin, have the potential of reducing sphincter tone by promoting smooth muscle relaxation at that level. If the outlet is already weak, incontinence can result.

Patients who are severely depressed may become incontinent because of inattention to basic functions such as toileting. Occasionally, a dependent patient with a passive-aggressive personality may feign incontinence, using it as an attention-getting device. Neither factor was thought to be operating in this depressed, but otherwise motivated patient. Tricyclic antidepressants, including desipramine, have anticholinergic activity and can paralyze the cholinergically active detrusor muscle and precipitate urinary retention with overflow incontinence. This generally occurs in elderly men with underlying prostatic enlargement, however, and the present patient had a residual urine of less than 30 cc. Anticholinergic agents can also cause urinary incontinence by promoting constipation and fecal impaction, resulting in urinary retention with overflow, or by causing confusional states which can lead to incontinence.

Hospitalization and institutionalization provide an inhospitable environment where independence and privacy are lacking. Patients are often required to urinate while recumbent, and are compelled to adhere to the staff's schedule rather than their own.   Such conditions are highly conducive to the development of urinary incontinence.

2. Nonpharmacologic measures are often the most effective way of dealing with urinary incontinence.   An essential measure is to seek out and reverse underlying causes of incontinence, such as offending medications, delirium, acute urinary tract infection, or polyuric states.   In established incontinence due to unstable bladder, bladder training should be instituted.   This consists of observing and recording the patient's micturition needs, and toileting at the longest possible interval (usually one-half to 2 hours) to keep the patient dry.   If continence is maintained for 48 hours, the interval can be lengthened.   This method is repeated until a reasonable goal is achieved, such as 4 hours of continence.   Pelvic floor exercises (contracting perineal muscles) with increasing numbers of repetitions should be instituted in cooperative female patients with outlet weakness, and may be highly effective.   In severe cases, surgical "sling" procedures should be considered.   If surgery is not an option, a vaginal pessary may be inserted to increase the vesico-urethral angle and support the pelvic floor.   The pessary is an oval-shaped coil that must be removed and cleaned at least once a month, or incarceration may occur.   Use of vaginal estrogen cream facilitates insertion and removal of the pessary.

If incontinence is not eradicated by other interventions, incontinence pads and garments can be used, but must be changed at appropriate intervals in immobilized patients so that psychologic harm, skin irritation, and decubitus ulcers do not result.   Many effective commercially available products are now available with varying capacity.

3. Pharmacologic treatment of unstable bladder consists of giving agents with anticholinergic or direct smooth muscle relaxant properties (antispasmodics). These agents relax the detrusor muscle and promote urine storage.   Popular antispasmodics include oxybutynin and flavoxate.   Propantheline, an antimuscarinic agent with antispasmodic action, may also be effective.   The tricyclic antidepressant, imipramine, has potent anticholinergic effect.   In addition, it prevents the reuptake of norepinephrine, resulting in stimulation of alpha-adrenergic receptors at the base of the bladder and increasing outlet resistance.   A switch from desipramine, which is weakly anticholinergic, to imipramine might be a useful move in this patient who has tolerated her other tricyclic well.   Both propantheline and imipramine are ganglionic blockers and may cause orthostatic hypotension.

Urethral resistance can be increased by imipramine.   Sympathomimetic agents such as phenylpropanolamine can do this as well, but may raise blood pressure.   Sympathomimetic agents can be combined with antispasmodics or with topical or systemic estrogen.   Estrogen may increase the tone of the estrogen-depleted urethra, and may also increase the sensitivity of alpha receptors to the effects of concurrently administered sympathomimetics.

The efficacy of pharmacologic therapy is far from guaranteed. Any pharmacologic agent is more likely to be effective when incontinence is mild to moderate, and unlikely to be effective in severe cases.

4. If aggressive measures in the nursing home are effective in keeping the patient dry, she might be able to go home. Unfortunately, they were not. Incontinence garments are not effective for more than a few hours, and it would be cruel and unhealthy to keep this alert patient in bed all day. She was unable to lose weight, as one would predict in an elderly, immobile, depressed, chronically obese patient. Neither rehabilitation nor maximum analgesic and anti-inflammatory medication strengthened her knee enough to make much difference, and knee surgery is not an option in a hemiparetic patient. She continued to require two-person assistance.

Families are often able to care for elderly parents at home, even when the work is considerable, but dealing with incontinence seems to be very problematic and is often a "last straw" in the family's ability or desire to take care of someone at home. Medicare pays little or nothing in the way of longterm chronic home care. Since the patient's financial needs are calculated without consideration of her children's income, the patient could "spend down" to the poverty level and qualify for Medicaid (Federal program for the poor, known by various names), which will pay for a good deal of home attendant services. However, no third-party payor will pay for two home attendants. The second home attendant would have to be paid for privately by the family, a situation that Medicaid would justifiably view with suspicion. The family could barely afford one 12-hour attendant, let alone two, and the only solution they could envision was that the patient's daughter would have to quit her job and assist in the care. The family could not afford this solution either, and the patient stayed in the nursing home. She soon "spent down," and Medicaid payments covered the cost. Fortunately, she grew accustomed to her environment, the family continued to visit regularly, and all involved became relatively comfortable with the solution.

Pearls:

1. Determination of residual urine is a simple test that can aid in the diagnosis and treatment of urinary incontinence. The patient is instructed to empty the bladder. Immediately after, a straight catheter is inserted and the remaining urine measured. Greater than roughly 75 to 100 cc is considered suspicious of urinary retention. Such patients should have further urologic evaluation before medical therapy is instituted.

2. In the overwhelming majority of cases, elderly American widows who live at home with a caregiver live with their eldest daughter. The caregiver of elderly men, in most cases, is the wife.

3. As many as 50% of older women have chronic asymptomatic bacteriuria, with or without pyuria. If such patients have chronic incontinence, it should not be attributed to an infected urinary tract, and antibiotic treatment neither eradicates the bacteriuria permanently nor does it cure the incontinence. Acute urinary tract infections, however, may precipitate reversible incontinence in patients with otherwise compensated bladder problems. In these cases, antibiotic treatment may restore continence.

Pitfalls:

1. Indwelling urethral or suprapubic catheters are not indicated in the treatment of chronic urinary incontinence except that due to intractable urinary retention. Catheters that remain in place for 7 days or more are associated with a 100% rate of urinary tract infection, which no measures can prevent or completely eradicate. Indwelling catheters or intermittent catheterization may be indicated for short-term use in incontinent patients with severe multiple decubitus ulcers until healing is established.

2. Uncomplicated cystocele causes modest urinary retention, not incontinence, unless the cystocele is large enough to cause obstruction with overflow incontinence.

3. Diabetic cystopathy is an autonomic neuropathy that causes an atonic bladder with urinary retention. It affects many patients with longstanding type I diabetes who have other signs of autonomic neuropathy. Most elderly diabetics have type II diabetes and if they have urinary incontinence, it is generally on another basis.

4. Anticholinergic effects are poorly tolerated by the elderly and are often the limiting factor in medical treatment of incontinence. Another problem is that medical treatment is usually useful only for mild to moderate symptoms.

References:

Burgio KL, Burgio LD. Behavior therapies for urinary incontinence in the elderly. Clin Geriatr Med 1986;2:809-827.

Resnick NM, Baumann MM. Incontinence in the nursing home patient. Clin Geriatr Med 1988;4:549-570.

Warren J. Catheters and catheter care. Clin Geriatr Med 1986;2:857-871.

Williams ME. Urinary incontinence in the elderly. Ann Intern Med 1982;97:895-907.

Hypertension

Case 17. A 75-year-old man has a blood pressure of 180/70. He is currently taking chlorthalidone 50 mg, clonidine 0.2 mg b.i.d., and potassium. He appears robust and has no complaints, except for pain in his calves when he walks. He has stable angina for which he takes occasional nitroglycerine. Physical examination reveals absent pedal pulses, but is otherwise normal. Pulse is 60 and regular.

Clue:

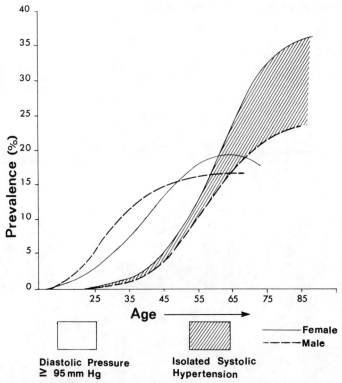

Adapted from Hutchison B. Hypertension in the elderly. Can Fam Phys 1981;27:1579-86; Wilking SVB, Belanger A, Kannel WB, et al. Determinants of isolated systolic hypertension. JAMA 1988;260:3451-3455.

Questions:

1. What is the significance of this patient's blood pressure?

2. What is the goal in managing his hypertension?

3. What treatments or medications are indicated for his blood pressure and what side effects can be expected?

4. What can be done for his claudication?

Answers:

1. Because this patient has systolic pressure greater than 160 and diastolic pressure lower than 90 mm Hg, he is said to have "isolated systolic hypertension" (ISH). This form of hypertension probably accounts for the vast majority of elevated blood pressure in the elderly population and is a different disorder than "essential" (systolic-diastolic) hypertension, in which diastolic pressure is 95 or more. ISH is probably due to age-related increase in stiffness and lack of distensibility of the arteries, a condition that occurs as a result of alterations of collagen and elastic tissue in the arterial media, accompanied by an increase in the calcium content of the arteries. Although elevated systolic pressure is associated with an increased risk of stroke, it is not known whether treatment of ISH reduces the risk. The age-related arterial changes that produce elevated blood pressure are widespread, and may contribute to in-situ problems in the cerebral vasculature itself. On the other hand, the geographic concentration of arteriosclerosis in vessels of the aortic arch tempts some investigators to relate this to a jet stream produced by high systolic pressures. Longitudinal studies are under way to determine the effects of treatment.

2. Because the risk-benefit ratio of treating ISH in the elderly is not known, geriatricians usually adopt the approach of lowering systolic blood pressure to roughly 160 mm Hg, as long as treatment does not produce symptoms. In extreme old age, the goal may be more conservative.

3. Salt restriction may be physiologically inappropriate in late life (see Case 1), particularly when salt-wasting diuretics are given. Other nonpharmacologic methods, such as weight loss, meditation, and biofeedback, may be tried but have not been systematically studied in elderly patients with ISH. Weight loss is difficult to attain in late life because of decreased physical activity and decreased metabolic rate.

    This nonobese man was put through a succession of medications and developed side effects on most of them. Clonidine produced dry mouth and worsened constipation. Dry mouth cannot be taken lightly in the elderly, who may have impaired salivary gland function and, if they wear dentures, may develop gingival irritation or ulceration. Beta blockers, which may be very well tolerated in older patients, should be selected carefully because of the increased susceptibility to heart failure, confusion, and bradycardia. On the other hand, beta blockers may fail to lower blood pressure more often in elderly than younger hypertensives, because of a decreased beta-receptor sensitivity that occurs with age. Beta blockers were tried because of the patient's angina, and pindolol was selected because its "intrinsic sympathomimetic activity" was expected to prevent further slowing of his heart rate. However, his claudication got worse, an effect that may have occurred because the beta blockade produced unopposed alpha stimulation and vasoconstriction. Calcium channel blocking agents are quite well tolerated, but nifedipine produced significant peripheral edema in this patient. The incidence of edema from nifedipine is said to be 10%, but the incidence is probably much higher in the elderly because of underlying venous insufficiency. All centrally acting agents may produce confusion in the elderly. Confusion is a common geriatric drug effect, but one that did not occur in this patient.

Hydralazine was given without adverse effects but did not lower the blood pressure. Reflex tachycardia, a noted side effect of this agent, is less common in the elderly because baroreflexes are often impaired or because sick sinus syndrome is present.

Like the majority of elderly patients, this man tolerated his diuretic well; however, many adamantly refuse diuretics if they exacerbate an underlying bladder problem. Hypokalemia from thiazide diuretics is common, and potassium depletion may increase cardiac arrhythmogenicity. Not atypically, this patient's serum potassium remained normal without supplements. Potassium-sparing diuretics need to be used with caution in the elderly because there is an increased tendency to develop hyperkalemia, which is thought to be due to age-related decrease in renin and aldosterone.

His blood pressure finally came under control with captopril, but potassium had to be discontinued when serum potassium level began to rise. Angiotensin converting enzyme inhibitors are well tolerated in elderly patients who do not have renal dysfunction. Labetolol, a beta blocker with alpha blocking activity, was added, and claudication did not worsen. In the elderly, labetolol may be more effective than simple beta blockers in controlling blood pressure because it overcomes the higher peripheral vascular resistance seen in elderly hypertensives.

4. Arterial claudication in the elderly is almost always due to progressive, diffuse arteriosclerosis, which is not amenable to surgical treatment. Medications known to exacerbate symptoms should be avoided. The xanthine, pentoxifylline (Trental), has been promoted for its ability to increase flexibility of the red cell, thereby reducing blood viscosity, but the drug has not been found to be particularly effective in clinical practice. The most sensible approach for this angina patient is a graded walking program in which he is instructed to walk through his leg pain, in order to stimulate the formation of collateral circulation. If pain is severe, analgesia can be given prior to his exercise. An exercise program has the additional benefit of counteracting the tendency for such patients to become sedentary, worsening their condition, reducing social contacts, and harming morale.

Pearls:

1. Intermittent claudication is almost always attributed to peripheral vascular disease, but in some cases can be due to lumbar spinal stenosis, a condition caused by narrowing of the lumbar spinal canal from osteoarthritis, degenerative disc disease, or spondylolisthesis. The absence of pedal pulses does not prove that symptoms are due to arterial disease. Spinal claudication is usually relieved temporarily by maneuvers that flex the lumbar spine, such as squatting or walking while leaning on a grocery cart or lawn mower. Laminectomy may eradicate this condition.

2. Preliminary evidence from Europe indicates that treatment of essential hypertension in the elderly reduces cardiovascular morbidity and mortality, but individuals over the age of 80 (a group composed mostly of women) do not achieve any benefit. The positive and negative data from this study cannot be extrapolated to ISH.

Pitfalls:

1. Overtreatment of hypertension in the elderly can result in a "hypotensive stroke." Cerebral autoregulation is impaired in old age, so that drops in peripheral arterial pressure may not be compensated readily in the cerebral circulation. Carotid or vertebral arteriosclerosis are often present and may exacerbate the problem. Ischemia in other organs may occur as well. Youthful goals of 120/80 are inappropriate for the elderly patient with hypertension.

2. Cuff pressure may indicate hypertension when actual intra-arterial pressure is normal, a situation referred to as "pseudohypertension." A clinical maneuver developed by Osler may be useful when a discrepancy is suspected. The radial artery is palpated and the blood pressure cuff inflated to systolic pressure in order to eradicate the pulse. If the artery is still palpable at this point, it is likely that the artery is stiff enough to produce a cuff pressure that is significantly higher than intra-arterial pressure. Occasionally, cuff pressure may be markedly higher, but this is generally seen in patients whose brachial arteries are severely calcified "pipes."

3. There is no "antihypertensive of choice" in geriatric practice. The treatment regimen must be strictly individualized, taking into account the array of possible side effects.

References:

Amery A, Brixko R, Clement D, et al. Efficacy of antihypertensive drug treatment according to age, sex, blood pressure, and previous cardiovascular disease in patients over the age of 60, Lancet 1986;2:589-595.

Feldman RD, Limbird RE, Nadeau J, et al. Alterations in leukocyte beta-receptor affinity with aging. A potential explanation for altered beta-adrenergic sensitivity in the elderly. N Engl J Med 1984;310:815-819.

Hall S, Bartleson JD, Burton MO, et al. Lumbar spinal stenosis. Ann Intern Med 1985;103:271-275.

Hutchison B. Hypertension in the elderly. Can Fam Phys 1981;27:1579-1586.

Kannel WB, Wolf PA, McGee DL, Dawber TR, McNamara P, Castelli W. Systolic blood pressure, arterial rigidity, and risk of stroke. JAMA 1981;245:1225-1229.

Messerli FH, Ventura HO, Amodeo C.   Osler's maneuver and pseudohypertension. N Engl J Med 1985;312:1548-1551.

Rowe JW. Aging and renal function. In: Arieff Al, DeFronzo RA. Fluid electrolyte and acid-base disorders.   New York: Churchill Livingstone, 1985:1231-1246.

Wallin JD, Shah SV.   Beta-adrenergic blocking agents in the treatment of hypertension. Arch Int Med 1987;147:654-664.

Wilking SVB, Belanger A, Kannel WB, et al. Determinants of isolated systolic hypertension. JAMA 1988;260:3451-3455.

Wollner L, McCarthy ST, Soper NDW, et al. Failure of cerebral autoregulation as a cause of brain dysfunction in the elderly. Brit Med J 1979;1:1117-1118.

Occupational Deterioration

Case 18.   A 69-year-old woman has worked as a secretary for many years, and is about to become your patient.   You receive a call from a concerned supervisor at her place of employment that the patient is no longer functioning well at work, where she is responsible for typing, payroll function, and signing checks.   The office staff has been assisting her, but her function has deteriorated so much that action is called for.   The supervisor wants to know what to expect, and whether there is anything she can do to help.

On physical examination, the patient's face is expressionless.   She walks slowly, without swinging her arms, and has a slightly stooped posture.   She has a resting, to-and-fro tremor of both hands, and her lips and legs are noted to tremble slightly.   Upper extremeties exhibit increased tone, suggestive of muscle rigidity.   The patient says things are going well at work, but she appears and sounds depressed.   Medication has been prescribed for her condition, but she takes it erratically, saying she can't remember to take it so often.

The patient lives alone, is unmarried, and has no children or close friends.

Questions:

1. What disease is the patient suffering from?

2. Why might she be depressed?

3. What are some reasons that she is not functioning well at work?

4. What can be done to maximize her occupational function?

Answers:

1. The patient has classic Parkinson's disease (PD), characterized in her case by signs such as "pill-rolling" tremor, bradykinesia (slowness of movement), rigidity, and mask-like facies.

2. Depression is extremely common in PD, and occurs out of proportion both to the severity of the disease and to what would be expected in a degenerative disease. For this reason, depression has been thought to be an endogenous feature of PD, related to neurohormonal alterations, rather than a secondary phenomenon. In addition, antiparkinsonian medications, particularly preparations of levodopa, may be responsible. Of course, a reactive depression would be possible in someone whose occupational function was waning, especially when there is a lack of social support.

3. Bradykinesia refers not merely to slowness of gait, but to a generalized diminution in the rate and extent of movement. Certainly the manual dexterity of a typist-payroll worker could be impaired by the disease. Handwriting characteristically deteriorates and not only shows the signs of a tremor, but may diminish in size ("micrographia"). Generalized symptoms such as fatigue and weakness are common, and along with depression, would certainly impair her stamina. The voice may become soft, making it difficult for others to understand the patient. Slowness of verbal response may give the appearance of dementia when none exists. This, combined with drooling that affects some patients, mask-like facies, and other symptoms, may interfere with personal interactions in the work setting. Alzheimer-like dementia is common, if not universal, in the later stages of PD, but had not yet affected this patient.

4. Although the prognosis for her career is not good, maximization of the patient's medical regimen, combined with supportive therapy, perhaps in conjunction with the interested supervisor, may buy time until she grows to view her medical condition realistically and makes plans for her future care. This woman is very fortunate that she works in a situation where others are patient and willing to help.

She may need to take levodopa-carbidopa (Sinemet) every few hours in order to have uniform control of her symptoms throughout her working day. The addition of dopaminergic amantadine (Symmetrel), or the dopamine agonist bromocriptine (Parlodel), may further improve function. Perhaps the patient's supervisor would be willing to assist in reminding her to take her medications during the day, assuming the patient, who appears to be a rather isolated individual, would allow any intervention. Consistency with the medical regimen in the evening will be less important than during the day. Since exercise is important in maintaining function in the face of muscle rigidity, daily walks during lunchtime or coffee breaks might be suggested.

Pearls:

1. Levodopa (L-dihydroxyphenylalanine) is a naturally occurring amino acid that exerts its pharmacologic effect through its chief metabolite, dopamine. Since most ingested levodopa is rapidly converted to dopamine, which does not pass the blood-brain barrier, levodopa is given in combination with carbidopa, a peripheral inhibitor of this conversion. This combination enables more levodopa to pass into the brain before degradation, and its efficacy is enhanced. The combination is far better than levodopa alone, since the large dose of the latter required to deliver adequate dopamine to the brain is poorly tolerated by the gastrointestinal system.

2. The "on-off" phenomenon is a form of symptom fluctuation experienced by many patients with PD, particularly in the later stages. It is characterized by rapid improvement shortly after a dose of Sinemet is given ("on"), followed by rapid deterioration ("off") at unpredictable intervals. This may be more than an end-of-dose phenomenon, and it has been suggested that it is related to the rapid entry of dopamine into the brain that has lost the ability to store the substance; alternatively, it could be due to the production of toxic drug metabolites that are produced by the deranged neuronal environment in late PD.

Pitfalls:

1. Most antiparkinsonian drug treatment is palliative and does not slow the course of the disease, which eventually results in severe debility and dementia. However, recent evidence indicates that deprenyl may have some effect in delaying clinical progression. Deprenyl is a selective monoamine oxidase type B inhibitor, which augments the effect of levodopa while avoiding potential pressor reactions seen with nonselective agents.

2. Anticholinergic agents such as benztropine (Cogentin) and trihexyphenidyl (Artane), and the anticholinergic antihistamine diphenhydramine (Benadryl) are sometimes prescribed in order to reduce the functional excess of acetylcholine that is thought to occur in PD. Once the mainstay of therapy, anticholinergic agents have largely been supplanted by dopaminergic drugs, and are now used mainly as adjunctive therapy in stubborn symptoms such as tremor, to eradicate symptoms such as drooling, and in patients who cannot tolerate the other agents.

3. Idiopathic PD must be distinguished from Parkinson-like symptoms that can be produced by drugs with dopamine antagonist activity, such as haloperidol, phenothiazines, and metoclopramide. Drug-induced parkinsonism is usually, but not always, reversible if the offending agent is discontinued.

4. Dopaminergic agents may produce choreiform movements and psychiatric symptoms such as paranoia and hallucinations. These drug-related symptoms are generally reversible and tend to be dose-related, but may be more common in the late stages of the disease, implying underlying neuronal deterioration or buildup of toxic drug metabolites as an etiology.

5. Parkinsonian tremor must be distinguished from "benign essential tremor," a common geriatric condition. Essential tremor differs in that it may be familial, worsens with intention, and is not associated with symptoms of PD, such as rigidity or bradykinesia.

6. Transplantation of adrenal medullary tissue remains a controversial, experimental approach to the treatment of PD, the early claims of great success notwithstanding.

References:

Calne DB, Langston JW. Aetiology of Parkinson's Disease. Lancet 1983;2:1457-1459.

Cummings JL.   The dementias of Parkinson's Disease: prevalence, characteristics, neurobiology, and comparison with dementia of the Alzheimer type.   Eur Neurol 1988;28 (suppl 1):15-23.

Goetz CG, Olanow W, Koller WC, Penn RD, Cahill D, Morantz R. Multicenter study of autologous adrenal medullary transplantation to the corpus striatum in patients with advanced Parkinson's disease. N Engl J Med 1989;320:337-341.

Lees AJ. L-Dopa treatment and Parkinson's Disease. Q J Med 1986;59:535-547.

Lieberman AN. Update in Parkinson disease. N Y State J Med 1987;87:147-153.

Parkes JD. Adverse effects of antiparkinsonian drugs. Drugs 1981;21:341-353.

Peterson DI, Price ML, Small CS. Autopsy findings in a patient who had an adrenal-to-brain transplant for Parkinson's Disease.   Neurology 1989;39:235-238.

Walton JN. Brain's disease of the nervous system. 8th ed. New York: Oxford University Press, 1977:579-600.

Leg Ulcer

<u>**Case 19.**</u> An 85-year-old man develops a leg ulcer. He has congestive heart failure, history of a stroke with residual weakness in his left hand and leg, and history of a fractured right hand. Topical treatment and leg elevations are prescribed, but a month later, his ulcer is much worse. The patient, who lives in a single room occupancy hotel (SRO), cannot care for his ulcer adequately because of poor manual dexterity and difficulty transferring between chair and bed. He refuses to hire a home attendant or nurse to give him daily care because he says he cannot afford it, but he does not qualify for Medicaid, which would pay for such services. You advise temporary hospitalization, noting that Medicare would pay, but he refuses, fearing that his color television, his most prized possession, would be stolen.

<u>**Clue:**</u>

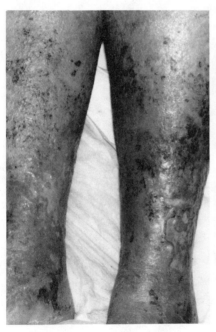 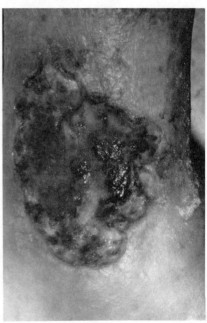

Questions:

1. Is the patient competent to refuse hospitalization?

2. What is happening to the patient's leg?

3. What care is recommended?

4. What are the consequences of improper care of the leg?

Answers:

1. The patient's mental status was normal, or at least normal enough, that he was competent to make the decision to refuse care of this curable condition. From a legal point of view, an individual is deemed competent until proven otherwise, and if physicians or caregivers disagree with this patient's decision, and feel strongly about his lack of competence, they would have to prove his incompetence before a judge and obtain a court order for hospitalization. Determination of competency is specific to the situation and is a determination that can be made by a lay person, namely, a judge who is not a physician. In actual practice, if a court order is sought, an experienced clinician, such as a psychiatrist, examines the patient and testifies regarding his ability to be making medical decisions. It is possible for someone who is partly impaired to be considered competent to refuse treatment--for example, someone who has psychotic hallucinations may still have the capacity to assess a medical situation if the psychotic ideation does not interfere with that assessment. In the present case, the medical personnel felt the patient was competent and reluctantly agreed to abide by his decision.

2. The patient has severe venous stasis, complicated by the edema of congestive heart failure, and resulting in an infected leg ulcer, stasis dermatitis, and a small area of cellulitis. Venous stasis alone produces edema and extravasation of blood with petechiae. In longstanding cases, fibrosis, nonpitting edema, and hyperpigmentation from hemosiderin deposition occur. Stasis dermatitis with erythema, scaling, and edema can be superimposed, and can resemble or be complicated by cellulitis.

3. Avoidance of trauma may prevent ulceration. Treatment consists of diuretics, leg elevation, debridement of necrotic tissue, and, if cellulitis is present, antibiotics. Stasis dermatitis should be treated with application of a moderate potency topical steroid, such as triamcinolone 0.1%. If arterial circulation is adequate, edema can also be managed with extrinsic pressure from a pressure stocking (Jobst) or 10- to 15-cm-wide elastic (Ace) bandage. Once debrided of necrotic tissue and exudate, the ulcer should be covered by an occlusive dressing. Occlusive dressings, like the roof of a blister, keep the wound moist and have been found to be at least as effective as permeable dressings that allow the wound to dry. Wound fluid has intrinsic healing capabilities, containing enzymes produced by white blood cells and bacteria, which digest necrotic tissue and fight infection. A commercially available hydrocolloid occlusive dressing (DuoDerm) forms a gel as the wound heals, allows granulation to occur, and, when removed, does not damage new epithelium. This type of dressing can be kept on for days, reduces nursing time, and is ideal for patients who cannot do wound care themselves. The

Unna boot, a zinc oxide, glycerine, and gelatine bandage, is molded and is kept on for a week, keeps the wound clean, and promotes drying, but has lost popularity to commercial occlusive and semi-occlusive dressings, which are easier to apply. If specialized dressings are not available, traditional treatment with daily cleansing and clean gauze dressing are highly effective. It is the quality and regularity of care that determine the outcome. Very large ulcers may require skin grafting.

Wound culture is generally not revealing, since skin ulcers are "dirty wounds" that are colonized by many species of bacteria. However, topical or oral antibiotics may sometimes be required.

4. If a leg ulcer is not adequately cared for, it may increase in diameter and depth.   Advanced cellulitis and even sepsis may occur.   Gangrene and amputation are rare in venous disease that is not complicated by arterial insufficiency.

There are many patients like the present one, who are unable to pay for home care, and proper treatment does not ensue until the medical condition becomes so serious that hospitalization is required. In this case, the situation went even beyond that stage before the patient agreed to hospitalization. The hospital would not allow him to bring his color television, and it was stolen, as he predicted.

Pearls:

1. A key feature that distinguishes a venous stasis ulcer from an arterial ulcer is the location, the latter occurring distally, in the toe or foot, the former occurring in the malleolar area, usually on the medial aspect. Venous ulcers usually are accompanied by other signs of chronic stasis, and arterial ulcers are generally more painful unless accompanied by severe peripheral neuropathy. Mixed pathology is common in geriatric patients.

2. Although leg ulcers are occasionally due to autoimmune disease, tumors, or infection with unusual microorganisms, 90% are due to venous stasis, and most of the remainder to arteriosclerotic or diabetic arterial disease.

Pitfalls:

1. Patients may have the unvoiced concern that a leg ulcer means that they are "going to lose the leg." This fear may cause them to resist hospitalization. A patient with a venous ulcer uncomplicated by ischemia of arterial insufficiency can be reassured that the condition is curable by proper medical care, and, on the average, heals within 6 weeks. In arterial insufficiency, proper treatment of ischemic ulcers can also prevent loss of limbs.

2. For leg elevation to be effective, there must be actual venous return, and the foot should be kept higher than the right atrium. If this cannot be achieved in chairs that are available in the home, the patient should be instructed to rest in bed or on a spacious couch with the foot elevated on pillows. Since complete bed rest is not always possible, or desirable, pressure stockings or a leg wrap with an Ace bandage can be used during the day, and the patient should be instructed to keep the legs moving when up. Unfortunately, many elderly are unable to put on tight elastic stockings or leg wraps.

If a prolonged period of bed rest is anticipated, anticoagulation should be given to patients considered at high risk of thrombophlebitis.

3. A patient's competence to make medical decisions is often taken for granted until he or she disagrees with the physician's recommendations. It is incumbent upon the physician to question whether the disagreement is a result of a failure to communicate with the patient, the physician's overconfidence in his or her opinion, or the patient's earnest wishes to forego a procedure deemed medically indicated.

References:

Agate JN. Aging and the skin--pressure sores. In: Brocklehurst JC, ed. Textbook of geriatric medicine and gerontology, 3rd ed. Edinburgh: Churchill Livingstone, 1985:915-934.

Marsh FH. Informed consent and the elderly patient. Clin Geriatr Med 1986;2:501-512.

Witkowski JA, Parish LC. Cutaneous ulcer therapy. Int J Dermatol 1986;25:420-426.

Change in Mental Status

<u>Case 20.</u> An 80-year-old nursing home patient is noted to be drowsy and confused. Blood pressure is 120/80. Pulse is 72 and regular. The nurse reports that the patient is "afebrile." Over the next few hours, the patient becomes stuporous and cannot be aroused. Blood pressure is 80/60, and pulse is 50 and regular. Rectal temperature is reported to be 95°F. She is transferred to the hospital.

The patient suffered a stroke 2 years ago, which left her with hemiplegia, severe aphasia, and dementia. She lives in a well-run nursing home. She spends most of her day seated in a wheelchair, or sitting in a chair by the window of her room. It happens to be New Year's Day, and staffing in the nursing home has been a little low.

She takes no medication, and is seen by her physician on a monthly basis in compliance with state and Federal requirements.

<u>Clue:</u>

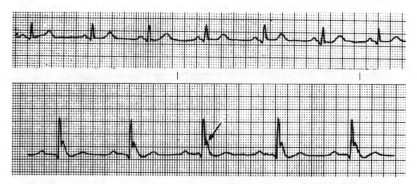

<u>Questions:</u>

1. What is delirium and what are its causes in the elderly? In this patient?

2. What are the risk factors that have caused her problem?

3. How might the patient's problem have been prevented?

Answers:

1. Delirium is an acute change in mental status, characterized by decreased attention span and alteration in the state of consciousness, resulting in disorientation and memory impairment. It is produced by an underlying organic disorder, and, in the elderly, a large number of conditions may be responsible. In addition to direct insults to the central nervous system, such as stroke, subdural hematoma, or encephalitis, systemic conditions produce acute confusional states more readily in the elderly than in the young. Common causes range from fecal impaction and urinary tract infection, to pneumonia and full-blown sepsis; metabolic derangements such as hypo- or hyperglycemia, electrolyte disturbances, or thyroid disease; drugs, particularly sedative-hypnotics, antidepressants, anticholinergic agents, centrally acting antihypertensives, and histamine-2 blockers, and such underrecognized offenders as indomethacin, isoniazid, and digoxin. In geriatric practice, any drug or systemic disease is suspect.

On admission to the hospital, this patient was found to have a temperature of 86°F, using a rectal probe thermometer. Hypothermia may itself produce delirium, but slow passive rewarming with blankets and warmed intravenous fluids produced no improvement in her mental status for 24 hours. At that point, laboratory results were reported and revealed that she was profoundly hypothyroid (T_4 = 0.8 μg/dL [N = 6.2-13.2] and TSH = 80 μU/mL [N = 0.8-4.8]). It was noted that, although her room in the nursing home seemed well-heated, the ambient temperature next to the window, where she spent much of her day, was quite low. The final diagnosis was myxedema, complicated by accidental hypothermia. Low ambient temperature and underlying hypothyroidism may have acted in concert to produce hypothermia.

2. In late life, there may be diminished perception of cold and abnormalities in thermoregulation. Impaired thermoregulation may be due to peripheral mechanisms (shivering and vasoconstrictor response), and central ones. Immobilized patients, such as the present one, do not generate heat through physical activity. Stroke itself may produce hypothalamic alterations in thermoregulation. Even if cold is perceived, disabled individuals may not be able to warm themselves adequately on their own, or to seek help. Hypothyroidism is an additional risk factor for hypothermia.

3. A policy of screening patients for thyroid disease on admission would probably have revealed hypothyroidism in this patient 2 years before. High-risk patients, such as the present one, do not require extremely low temperatures or prolonged exposure to the cold, but may develop hypothermia in cases of sudden changes in temperature or in conditions of temperature fluctuation. She may have had impaired cold perception, and could not

complain or produce adequate heat endogenously. Dependent elderly patients must be protected from large temperature fluctuations since they cannot protect themselves. Caregivers of home-bound elderly should visit frequently and see that these people are warm enough in winter, and cool enough in the summer.

Pearls:

1. Hypothermia may depress the myocardium and the conducting system, producing arrhythmias and cardiac failure. Characteristic findings on the electrocardiogram include fine baseline oscillations, prolonged P-R interval, and "J" (Osbourne) wave, a small deflection seen in conjunction with the QRS complex, early in the ST segment. The J wave is seen in fewer than 50% of hypothermia patients, is present more often in severe degrees of hypothermia, and disappears on rewarming. Its origin is a subject of debate. The irregular baseline is felt to be produced by increased muscle tone and subtle tremor that accompany hypothermia.

2. Abnormalities in thermoregulation put the elderly at risk for heat stroke as well. Hot, humid weather and enclosed apartments without adequate air circulation may lead to heat stroke in elderly people, even in the absence of physical exertion.

Pitfalls:

1. Ordinary thermometers do not record temperatures below 94°F, and, as might have been the case here, are often not shaken down even to that level when temperature is taken. If hypothermia is suspected, a special thermometer must be used.

2. Although the causes of dementia and delirium overlap, and the syndromes may coexist, they are distinct. Dementia is characterized by memory loss and impairment of higher intellectual function, but the state of consciousness is not altered, and the patient, though confused, is alert. In delirium, memory loss and intellectual impairment are secondary features resulting from global impairment in the central nervous system. Dementia is generally insidious in onset, slowly progressive, and most often due to irreversible causes. Delirium is generally acute or subacute in onset, and, depending on etiology, may progress to coma; more often than not, it is due to a potentially reversible condition. Acute mental status change in a cognitively normal or demented patient is due to a new, underlying medical condition, and constitutes a medical emergency.

References:

American Psychiatric Association.   Diagnostic and statistical manual of mental disorders (DSM-III-R). Washington, D.C., 1987:100-107.

Besdine RW.   Dementia and delirium.   In: Rowe JW, Besdine RW, eds. Geriatric Medicine. 2nd ed. Boston: Little, Brown, 1988:375-401.

Desforges ZJ. Delirium in the elderly.   N Engl J Med 1989;320:528-582.

Reuler JB. Hypothermia: pathophysiology, clinical settings, and management. Ann Intern Med 1978;89:519-527.

Trevino A, Razi B, Beller BM.   The characteristic electrocardiogram of accidental hypothermia.   Arch Int Med 1971;127:470-473.

Annual Physical

Case 21.　An 84-year-old widow lives alone in her apartment in a "total care community" where payment includes full medical care. She is summoned to the medical clinic for her "annual physical."

The patient says she can't understand why she is there, because she feels "just fine." You explain the need for periodic health screening, doing so in a loud voice, since she has an obvious hearing loss. "You don't have to shout," she says, a little annoyed. "I'm not hard of hearing."

Physical examination reveals blood pressure of 140/80, pulse of 72 and regular. She appears robust and has a normal gait. Physical examination is completely normal, including breast, rectal, neurologic, and mental status examinations. Tympanic membranes are normal and well visualized. Stool is guaiac negative. She refuses pelvic examination, stating that she is "too old for that."

Clue:

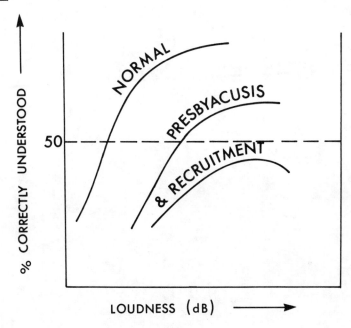

Questions:

1. Is the patient "hard of hearing" or not? What is going on?

2. What examinations would round out her annual physical?

3. What laboratory evaluations should she have as part of an accepted health screening program?

4. What immunizations are recommended?

Answers:

1. She is hard of hearing, as is obvious to the speaker but less so to the listener, a common inconsistency in the setting of progressive sensorineural hearing loss that occurs commonly in late life. This condition is referred to as "presbyacusis." Most people with presbyacusis will hear better when spoken to loudly, but if loud speaking is perceived as shouting, the patient might be experiencing the "recruitment phenomenon." People with normal hearing can hear and understand an increasing number of speech stimuli as the loudness is increased above a whisper (see Clue). With presbyacusis, there is a leveling off of the amount that can be heard as loudness increases. Thirty percent of people with presbyacusis experience the recruitment phenomenon, in which the amount that can be heard actually decreases as a particular state of loudness is reached. Such people have a great deal of difficulty being fitted with hearing aids, which amplify extraneous noise as well as sounds that the patient wants to hear. The best approach is to speak distinctly, in an ordinary or slightly loud voice, looking directly at the patient.

2. Intraocular pressure should be measured annually (tonometry) since open angle glaucoma can remain asymptomatic for years and is a preventable cause of blindness.

Pelvic examination with pap smear should be done in all elderly women. Most of the older generation have not been adequately screened according to American Cancer Society (ACS) guidelines, and many have never had a pap smear or have not seen a gynecologist since menopause. The incidence of carcinoma-in-situ, detected by pap smear, decreases dramatically with age over 30, but the incidence of invasive cervical cancer increases with age. The ACS recommends that the interval between pap smears is left to the physician's discretion following "three or more consecutive satisfactory normal annual examinations," but because it is inexpensive and noninvasive, annual screening is often done, and is still recommended by the American College of Obstetricians and Gynecologists. Despite the high incidence of false negatives, many cases of endometrial cancer, a cancer of late life, can be detected on pelvic examination or pap smear. Periodic gynecologic evaluation also provides the opportunity to screen for vulvar and vaginal cancers, which, though rare, occur most often in the elderly.

3. Annual mammogram is recommended for all older women. The incidence of breast cancer increases with age. The American Cancer Society also recommends periodic sigmoidoscopy in people over 50, to screen for colon cancer. Blood tests should include complete blood count, primarily as a screen for colon cancer. Thyroid function tests should be performed because thyroid disease is difficult to diagnose on clinical grounds in the elderly. T_4 and T_3RU

are most cost-effective in large screening programs, but are not as sensitive as TSH in detecting early hypothyroidism.

4. Influenza vaccine should be given annually in late fall to all people over the age of 65. Although deaths that occur during influenza epidemics are often caused by viruses other than influenza virus, influenza is the only respiratory virus for which an effective vaccine exists, and when deaths occur, they are generally in people older than 65. Community-wide immunization is particularly important in closed communities where epidemics can be curtailed only when vaccine rate approaches 75%. Pneumococcal vaccine (Pneumovax) should be given to all people over 65 since the incidence of pneumococcal disease increases dramatically with age, with the elderly population experiencing the most severe disease and the greatest mortality. Pneumovax should be given only once since the incidence of local and systemic adverse effects is higher in patients given repeat doses. Tetanus and diphtheria are rare, but mortality and the most severe morbidity among adults occurs primarily in the under-immunized, older population. If immunization history is not known, or if a booster has not been given in the past 10 years, primary series should be given. Tetanus and diphtheria toxoid may be given alone, or together as the usual adult preparation (Td).

Pearls:

1. Audiologic evaluation consists of audiometry (pure-tone testing), and speech testing. Audiometry is performed by presentation of tones through the use of earphones, applying sounds of varying loudness in decibels and different frequencies (Hertz). In presbyacusis, high-frequency sounds are generally lost first. Speech testing consists of the delivery of monosyllabic words at a comfortable level of loudness, a level at which normal young people will understand 100% of what is heard. Certain patients may perform fairly well in audiometry but poorly on speech testing. Such patients are said to have problems with "discrimination" and often fail to distinguish between rhyming words with high frequency, voiceless consonants, such as "thin" and "shin," or "cap" and "tap."

2. A treatable form of hearing loss that occurs commonly in the elderly is impacted cerumen. With age, the glands that produce cerumen tend to produce a harder wax than previously. Complete occlusion may cause rapid onset of hearing loss, often unilateral, but can be remedied with irrigation of the external auditory canal or by extracting the wax.

Pitfalls:

1.   Automated chemistry testing is not a cost-effective health screen in asymptomatic elderly, and frequent abnormalities are detected, leading to expensive and potentially dangerous workups. In practice, however, automated chemistry is routine.

2.   Measurement of serum cholesterol is not a required part of health screening in people over 75, since the health benefits of lowering cholesterol in the elderly are not known. However, many people are curious about their cholesterol level and highly motivated to improve their health. Furthermore, an elevated cholesterol may be an added incentive for people to exercise and improve their diet. No action should be taken on an elevated cholesterol done without measurement of high and low density subfractions, since the predictive value of total cholesterol declines with age.

3.   Pneumovax is effective against 23 common strains of pneumococcus represented in the vaccine, but not against other strains. Moreover, high-risk, debilitated patients may not mount a sufficient antibody response to the vaccine. Still, the safety and efficacy of this agent justify its general use.

References:

American Cancer Society. Guidelines for the cancer-related checkup: recommendations and rationale. Ca-A Cancer J for Clinicians 1980;30(4):193-240.

American Cancer Society. Summary of current guidelines for the cancer-related checkup: recommendations, 1988.

Bentley DW. Immunizations in the elderly. Bull NY Acad Med 1987;63:533-551.

Fisch L. Special senses--the aging auditory system. In: Brocklehurst JC, ed. Textbook of geriatrics and gerontology, 3rd ed. Edinburgh: Churchill Livingstone, 1985:484-499.

Health and Policy Committee. American College of Physicians. Pneumococcal vaccine. Ann Intern Med 1986;104:118-120.

Simberkoff MS, Cross AP, Al-Ibrahim M, et al. Efficacy of pneumococcal vaccine in high-risk patients: results of a Veterans Administration cooperative study. N Engl J Med 1986;315:318-327.

Office Visit

Case 22. An 80-year-old woman lives in the same total care community as the patient in the previous case, and is summoned for her annual physical. She has been living there for just a year and greets you happily. She is "just thrilled" that you are a geriatric specialist, because there are a number of things she has been wanting to talk to you about.

She explains that she used to be "tall and slim, with a nice, flat tummy," but now her abdomen sticks out and she has trouble finding clothing to fit her, because of "that hump." She is annoyed that she is "covered with wrinkles," but knows she can't do anything about that. She is more concerned about her memory, which is not as good as it used to be, and would like to discuss this with you. She is socially and physically active, plays bridge every Wednesday evening, and goes for long walks, wearing her "Reeboks." She refuses to play shuffleboard because "that's for old people," and she thinks it's the "most boring game on earth." She reads the <u>Philadelphia Inquirer</u> avidly, and is distressed about "the Ayatollah and what he is doing to that poor writer. . . what's his name? See? I can't even remember his name!"

The patient has never smoked. A retired kindergarten teacher, she shares her apartment with her husband of 50 years. He is a retired engineer who is in relatively good health. They have no children.

The patient is robust, friendly, and cooperative. She leaps onto the examining table with great agility, still wearing her Reeboks. She appears to be a little hard of hearing, and she explains that she isn't wearing her hearing aid, which she refers to as "that awful thing." She has moderate kyphosis and a protruberant abdomen, her "bête-noir." Her blood pressure is 160/70, and her pulse is 64 and regular. Barefoot, she is 5 feet 3 inches tall and weighs 140 pounds. Her upper arms, she points out, are "flabby." She has "horrid brown things" (dark brown keratotic lesions that have a stuck-on appearance) covering her back and a few on her anterior thorax and under her breast. She has a bruit over her right carotid artery. There is a grade I/VI systolic ejection murmur heard best over the apex. The rest of the physical examination is normal.

Blood count and screening blood chemistries are normal, except for a serum calcium level of 11.4 mg/dL (N = 8.5-11.0). Her EKG shows normal sinus rhythm with a left axis deviation.

Clue:

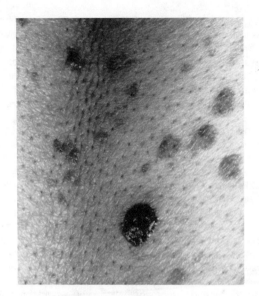

Questions:

1. How should you approach the problem of her

    a. skin lesions?
    b. serum calcium level?
    c. hearing problem?
    d. sagging skin?
    e. carotid bruit?
    f. heart murmur?

2. What should the patient be told about her
    a. figure problem?
    b. memory problem?
    c. electrocardiogram?

3. Why has she lost height?

4. At the age of 50 years, she was considered a slim 130 pounds. Should she now go on a diet?

Answers:

1. a. Her skin lesions are seborrheic keratoses. These are benign lesions, which increase in incidence with age. The etiology is not known. Since they are benign, they do not need to be removed unless the patient finds them cosmetically disagreeable. Individual lesions, strategically located, may become irritated when clothing or underwear rubs on them, and can be removed surgically or with electrodesiccation. Reassurance as to the benignity of seborrheic keratoses is called for.

b. Incidental finding of hypercalcemia on automated chemistry screening in elderly women is often due to asymptomatic, primary hyperparathyroidism (HPTH). There is great laboratory and diurnal variability in serum calcium measurements, so the test should be repeated on a fasting specimen. Drug inventory should be done to exclude the use of thiazide diuretics and calcium supplements, which can make HPTH biochemically manifest, and use of megadoses of vitamin D should be ruled out. If calcium is truly and spontaneously elevated, parathyroid hormone should be measured. If hyperparathyroidism is confirmed, chemistries should be followed and medical treatment with oral phosphates or estrogen should be considered. Surgical treatment is usually not warranted in asymptomatic states. Her kyphosis is most likely due to postmenopausal osteoporosis, but, if she proved to have HPTH and if there were no contraindication, she would be one of the few elderly women in whom treatment might be warranted for the prevention of further bone loss (see Case 15). Estrogen normalizes serum calcium and stabilizes bone changes in women with hyperparathyroidism.

Occult cancer is always a possibile explanation for hypercalcemia, but extensive workups in these situations are generally unwarranted.

c. The patient should be questioned as to why she is not using her hearing aid (amplification). Hearing aids of all varieties amplify not only what a person wishes to hear, but unwanted ambient noise as well, a situation that is often intolerable. Those who experience the recruitment phenomenon (see Case 21) may find this particularly annoying. Batteries must be changed frequently and impaired manual dexterity may hinder the ability to change the tiny battery and adjust the volume control. Many individuals dislike wearing a behind-the-ear hearing aid for cosmetic reasons. In-the-ear amplification may be a suitable alternative and should be considered in such patients. These cosmetically more acceptable hearing aids, unfortunately, do not fit if the external auditory canal is too small.

d. The patient's skin sags because of age changes in collagen and elastin. This process is irreversible, and to date, not preventable. Skin wrinkling is due largely to sunlight and other environmental ravages. This is termed "photoaging," or "extrinsic aging," and is to be distinguished from intrinsic aging of the skin. Life-long use of sun-blocking creams, avoidance of excessive sunlight exposure, and abstaining from smoking reduce the degree of skin wrinkling. Topical tretinoin (Retin-A) shows some promise in the treatment of fine wrinkling and other signs of photoaging, but it has not been studied in the elderly and its longterm toxicity is not known.

Skin dryness can be minimized with the use of emollient creams, and by reducing bathing time.

e. This patient has an asymptomatic carotid bruit, an incidental finding seen in more than 10% of people over 65. There is no convincing evidence that carotid endarterectomy or treatment with platelet inhibitors reduces the risk of transient ischemic attack or stroke in such patients. A nationwide study of asymptomatic carotid artery stenosis is underway.

f. Depending on the population studied, 30-60% of people over 65, and as many as 80% of people 80 years of age and older have heart murmurs. Systolic murmurs can be due to the same pathology seen in any age group, but are commonly due to sclerosis of a nonstenotic aortic valve, and may be heard in the "wrong location" because of the flow dynamics and because of alterations in thoracic geography. If the patient claims to be asymptomatic, careful history, physical evaluation, and electrocardiogram, CBC, and thyroid function tests usually are all that are required. Because potentially progressive lesions, such as aortic stenosis or septal hypertrophy may be present, followup is desirable.

2. a. The patient's abdomen may be protruding because of her kyphosis. If this is the case, the problem is not reversible, but she may wish to select figure-flattering clothing. Tight-fitting jackets and blouses are not designed for the kyphotic individual. Loose fitting tops may circumvent this problem. Abdominal tone can be maximized with isometric exercises. Sit-ups are to be discouraged in spinal osteoporosis because of the tendency to flex the thoracic spine. Erect posture and exercises that emphasize gentle thoracic extension are recommended.

b. Patients who complain that they have memory problems usually do not have dementia. Significant pathology is generally brought to a physician's attention by family members and not by patients themselves. This woman's obvious clarity of mind on the interview and her discussion of current events makes any pathology extremely unlikely. However, a simple, formal mental status examination should be considered because she will probably score well and gain some reassurance. The commonly used Mini-Mental State examination

(MMS), which tests orientation, memory, attention, and language, can be performed in 10 to 15 minutes, but a five-item version of the MMS may be at least as accurate in terms of sensitivity and specificity. This brief examination asks the day, month, and year; subtraction of serial 7's from 100 (five successive answers) or the spelling of "world" backwards; recalling three words after 5 minutes.

It is common for cognitively normal people to experience difficulty with name retrieval, even in early middle age. If this is her main problem, she can be reassured that she is not "getting senile."

c. She should be told that her EKG is normal for her age. Left axis deviation is the most commonly found "abnormality" in the elderly, but seen alone, has no prognostic significance.

3. She has lost height because of progressive kyphosis from wedging and compression of individual vertebrae. Other factors that contribute to age-related loss of height include decrease in the intervertebral disc spaces from desiccation of the nucleus pulposus and degeneration of the disc. There is also slight flexion at the knee and hip with age. All of these factors can lead to considerable loss of height over time.

4. Her current weight should be evaluated in light of the fact that she was once 5 foot 6 inches tall. It is inaccurate to assess obesity based on crown to floor measurements in the elderly. Arm span measurements, or tibial length are probably a better guide. Skinfold thickness can also be expected to be less accurate in the elderly because of increased skin laxity (the patient herself has made this observation). For clinical purposes, obesity can be judged by inspection. A modest increase in weight with age is considered normal, and is probably desirable, since it is associated with longevity in the nondiabetic, normotensive elderly.

Pearls:

1. Another common form of skin lesion that occurs in the elderly is the actinic ("senile," "solar") keratosis. Actinic keratoses are tan-colored, relatively flat, rough lesions that occur predominantly in sun-exposed areas, such as the forehead, dorsum of the hands, and shoulders, and are most common in fair-skinned people. These lesions should be removed because they occasionally progress to squamous carcinoma, although metastatic disease is unusual.

Actinic keratoses occur in up to 100% of Caucasian elderly studied, but are not a problem in black populations. Likewise, skin cancer is rare in blacks. Seborrheic keratoses, however, are common.

2. Basal cell carcinoma, which this patient does not have, is the most common tumor affecting light-skinned elderly.   It also is related to sunlight exposure and is increasing in frequency, but is of very low-grade malignancy and is sometimes referred to as "basal cell epithelioma." Although this tumor rarely metastasizes, it should be removed because it has a tendency to enlarge and erode adjoining structures.   Basal cell carcinoma is unusual in dark-skinned people.

Pitfalls:

1.   Minor cosmetic surgery, such as the removal of unwanted skin lesions, should not be discouraged in the elderly who desire such procedures. Cosmesis and good grooming are signs of good mental health, and should be encouraged.   On the other hand, it may be impractical to embark on a campaign to remove extensive lesions such as those in this patient.

2.   Seborrheic keratosis may resemble the nodular form of malignant melanoma, except that the latter tend to be more darkly pigmented and grow rather rapidly.   If there is any doubt as to the diagnosis, biopsy must be done.

3.   Hearing aids are very expensive and are not reimbursed by Medicare. Many states now require that patients be able to purchase a hearing aid trial for a modest amount, so that if they are not satisfied with the results, the apparatus can be returned.   Unfortunately, not all elderly are aware of this option, and it is not uncommon for an unscrupulous merchant to take advantage of this fact.

4.   Although sunlight exposure may produce skin lesions and extrinsic aging, avoidance of the sun can lead to vitamin D deficiency.   It is estimated that 15 minutes 2 to 3 times a week is all that is required for a light-skinned individual to achieve adequate vitamin D status.

References:

Andres R. Mortality and obesity: the rationale for age-specific height-weight tables. In: Andres R, Bierman EL, Hazzard WR, eds.   Principles of Geriatric Medicine. New York: McGraw-Hill, 1985:311-318.

Campbell A, Caird FI, Jackson TFM.   Prevalence of abnormalities of electrocardiogram in old people.   Brit Heart J 1974;36:1005-1011.

Duthie EH, Gambert SR, Tresch D.   Evaluation of the systolic murmur in the elderly. J Am Geriatr Soc 1981;29:498-502.

Fitzpatrick TB, Eisen AZ, Wolff K, Freedberg IM, Austen RF, eds. Dermatology in general medicine. 3rd ed. New York: McGraw-Hill, 1987:733-765.

Folstein MF, Folstein SE, McHugh PR. "Mini-Mental State," a practical method for grading the cognitive state of patients for the clinician. J Psychiatr Res 1975;12:189-198.

Gilchrest BA. Age-associated changes in the skin. J Am Geriatr Soc 1982;30:139-143.

Howell TH. Cardiac murmurs in old age: a clinico-pathological study. J Am Geriatr Soc 1967;15:509-516.

Klein LE, Roca RP, McArthur J, et al. Diagnosing dementia: univariate and multivariate analyses of the mental status examination. J Am Geriatr Soc 1985;33:483-488.

Marcus R, Madvig P, Crim M, Pont A, Kosek J. Conjugated estrogens in the treatment of postmenopausal women with hyperparathyroidism. Ann Intern Med 1984;100:633-640.

Tindall JP. Skin changes and lesions in our senior citizens: incidences. Cutis 1976;18:359-362.

Weiss JS, Ellis CN, Headington JT, et al. Topical tretinoin improves photoaged skin. A double-blind vehicle-controlled study. JAMA 1988;259:527-532.

"Mother is not herself"

Case 23. A 78-year-old Causasian woman with a history of left hip fracture develops intermittent pain in her right buttock and is told that she has sciatica. Her fracture had been repaired with an Austin-Moore hemiprosthesis but she developed acetabular erosion and now has degenerative arthritis of the joint. She has been treated with a variety of nonsteroidal anti-inflammatory agents for her pains and ambulates with difficulty, using a cane. She now complains that she has been feeling weak and has "pains all over." Her daughter, who accompanies her to your office, says her mother is "not herself." She is depressed, not eating, and complains all the time of "one thing or another. . . aches, pains, headaches, you name it."

On physical exam, the patient is of average build and has a depressed affect. She has slight kyphosis and there is decreased range of motion of her left hip. The left leg is slightly shorter than the right. There is questionable tenderness of the right buttock in the distribution of the sciatic nerve. Proximal muscle weakness is demonstrated in the upper and, to a lesser extent, the lower extremities, although the patient does not appear to be making a true effort on testing. Her upper arms are tender when squeezed. The remainder of the physical examination is within normal limits.

Blood tests are ordered and the patient is instructed to return in a week, but the daughter wants to take her mother to Florida so she "can get over this depression." Desipramine 25 mg is prescribed in an effort to treat the depressive symptoms and the chronic pains, and the patient is urged to contact a doctor in Florida.

Six weeks later you receive a long-distance call from the patient's daughter, who reports that her mother suddenly developed a serious symptom the night before. Until that time she was clinically unchanged.

Clue:

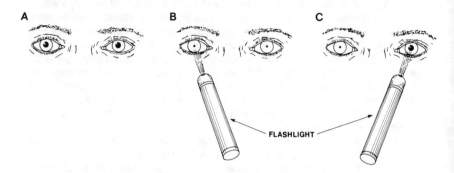

Questions:

1. What serious problem might have developed, taking the patient's other symptoms into account?

2. What should be done?

3. What will be the result?

Answers:

1. The patient's aches and pains, weakness, muscle tenderness, headaches, and depression were all strongly suggestive of polymyalgia rheumatica (PMR), a nonspecific syndrome that often culminates in temporal arteritis. It is common for PMR to be diagnosed as depression, or to be overlooked if the symptoms are mingled with other rheumatologic problems. An alarming event that prompts the patient to seek immediate help is sudden visual loss due to temporal arteritis involving branches of the ophthalmic artery. Occlusion of the posterior ciliary artery, which nourishes the optic nerve head, has produced ischemic optic neuropathy and unilateral visual loss in this patient. In addition to typical funduscopic findings of disc edema and pallor, this patient has a "Marcus-Gunn pupil": the direct light reflex of the involved eye is absent, but the pupil reacts consensually to light. When light is shone into the intact eye both pupils constrict (B); when light is quickly shifted to the diseased eye, the pupil appears to be dilating in response to light (C). Impulses travel via the intact optic nerve to the central nervous system and crossed fibers produce consensual constriction in the diseased eye via the intact efferent limb, the oculomotor nerve. The Marcus-Gunn pupil is not specific for temporal arteritis, but may be demonstrated in other conditions that damage the optic nerve.

This patient was also found to have tender, palpable temporal arteries, making the diagnosis of temporal arteritis a virtual certainty.

The blood tests that had been done before she left for Florida were normal except for an erythrocyte sedimentation rate (ESR) of 98 mm/hr, hemoglobin of 11.2 g/dL, and elevated serum globulins, findings typical of this disease. When elderly people present with nonspecific symptoms, often summarized in phrases such as, "my mother is not herself," full evaluation and followup are required.

2. Because of the danger of damage to the other eye, steroids need to be started immediately. On the basis of the history obtained over the phone, the patient should be instructed to go to a local emergency room if a physician is not otherwise available. The original physician should establish telephone contact and report the earlier findings. The recommended starting dose of prednisone for temporal arteritis is 60-80 mg per day; tapering may be started when reversible symptoms are gone and when sedimentation rate is normal or reaches a plateau.

There is much debate as to the necessity of a temporal artery biopsy, which, if positive, often reveals granulomatous arteritis with giant cells, but smooth muscle necrosis, destruction of internal elastic membrane, intimal fibrosis, or nonspecific inflammation may be present or dominate. If the presentation includes the classic tender, swollen temporal artery, greatly elevated ESR, and dramatic response to steroids, many argue that a biopsy would not change the treatment and need not be done. Conversely, biopsy may be negative. However, if there is any doubt as to the diagnosis (e.g., a normal ESR or sudden visual loss without systemic symptoms), a biopsy should be done. Temporal artery biopsy is a benign office procedure, while adverse effects of steroids in the elderly may be particularly severe, and consigning someone to indefinite treatment when the diagnosis is uncertain may produce a therapeutic predicament when side effects begin to occur. Negative biopsy should not deter treatment if clinical suspicion is strong.

If the patient had PMR without temporal arteritis, the symptoms would quickly resolve on only 10-15 mg of prednisone per day. Once symptoms of PMR are controlled, aspirin or nonsteroidal anti-inflammatory agents may be adequate in some patients and steroids can be withdrawn, although this does not guarantee that symptoms will not recur in the future.

3. Treatment is likely to reduce or eliminate systemic symptoms such as pains, weakness, and depression, within a day or two. This relief is quite dramatic, and persistence of symptoms should put the diagnosis in doubt. In elderly people, it is not uncommon for some symptoms to persist if they are due to unrelated pathology. In this case, the patient continued to have left hip pain from sequelae of her fracture, and right buttock pain, which was due to sciatica from coexistent degenerative disc disease ("osteoarthritis of the spine"). Sometimes (but by no means always) there is a partial or complete return of vision that is either spontaneous, the result of treatment, or due to the fact that temporal arteritis may produce typical transient ischemic attacks. This patient had some return of vision and dramatic relief of all of her systemic symptoms, and became "a new person." ESR, serum globulins, and hemoglobin normalized.

Symptoms may be completely and permanently eradicated, but, off steroids, many patients develop recurrent symptoms, some after many years. Once asymptomatic, patients should have periodic determination of ESR, and should be treated if ESR starts to rise.

Pearls:

1. PMR is much less common in the black population than in nonblacks. The reasons for this are not known.

2. Autopsy studies have revealed histopathologic changes in medium- and large-sized arteries throughout the body, although clinical manifestations are generally absent. Involved arteries outside the head and neck may include brachial, aortic arch, abdominal aorta, femoral, and mesenteric.

3. A positive "kiss sign" is pathognomonic for PMR and temporal arteritis. The kiss sign is positive if, 24 hours after you start the patient on steroids, she throws her arms around you and says, "Oh, doctor! I feel so much better, I could kiss you!" This feature has not been studied in a controlled fashion, but has been vouched for by such geriatric rheumatologists as its describer, Dr. Irving Karten, and verified by myself.

Pitfalls:

1. Morning stiffness is a common complaint in PMR, may be severe, and is similar to that which occurs in rheumatoid arthritis. If typical rheumatoid joint findings are present, however, the patient does not have PMR but may have a PMR-like syndrome that is seen in other collagen-vascular diseases.

2. Presentations may include jaw claudication, respiratory symptoms, fever of unknown origin, ear pain, hoarseness, stroke, and other symptoms attributed to inflammatory changes in medium- and large-sized arteries anywhere in the body. These symptoms are not necessarily accompanied by typical systemic or classic localized symptoms. There should always be a high index of suspicion if an elderly person develops peculiar symptoms that are not explained by other pathology.

3. The elderly suffer the same spectrum of adverse effects from steroids as do younger adults, but, because of underlying pathology, older patients are particularly vulnerable to side effects such as osteoporosis, acceleration of cataracts, leg edema, diabetes, and increased intraocular pressure.

4. ESR is not always elevated in temporal arteritis (see Problem 6, Part II).

References:

Chuang T, Hunder GG, Ilstrup DM, et al. Polymyalgia rheumatica: a 10 year epidemiologic and clinical study. Ann Intern Med 1982;97:672-680.

Hall S, Lie JT, Kurland LT, et al. The therapeutic impact of temporal artery biopsy. Lancet 1983;2:1217-1220.

Healey LA. The spectrum of polymyalgia rheumatica. Clin Geriatr Med 1988;4:323-331.

Huston KA, Hunder GG, Lie JT. Temporal arteritis: a 25-year epidemiologic, clinical, and pathologic study. Ann Intern Med 1978:162-167.

Wong RL, Korn JH.   Temporal arteritis without an elevated erythrocyte sedimentation rate.   Am J Med 1986;80:959-964.

"Mother is breathing funny"

Case 24. An 82-year-old woman resides in a nursing home. She has suffered a major hemispheric stroke and has severe global aphasia and right hemiplegia. Her daughter visits regularly. One day, the daughter reports that her mother is "breathing funny."

You are very busy writing monthly notes on several other nursing home patients, but you enter the patient's room and note that she does not appear to be in respiratory distress. Her pulse feels normal. On physical examination, she appears in her usual state. She is lying in bed, staring into space. Breath sounds are not well heard, the examination of the lungs being limited by the patient's inability to cooperate fully. You listen patiently, and breath sounds become fuller. Coarse crepitations are heard at both bases, unchanged from previous examinations. There is a harsh systolic ejection murmur heard over the right sternal border. Her hemiplegic extremities are moderately edematous, but there is no pitting, and this finding is unchanged from previous examinations. There is no edema on the left. You ask the nurse to check her vital signs while you complete the paper work. A few moments later the nurse finds you and tells you with alarm that the patient is breathing at a rate of 40 breaths per minute. Her blood pressure is 120/70 and her pulse is 68 and regular. You run to the room and find the patient lying with her eyes closed, not breathing.

Questions:

1. What should you do next?

2. What is causing this problem?

3. Why are other signs of the patient's underlying condition absent? What other clues can you seek?

4. What should you do now?

Answers:

1. You should observe the patient for a moment more. She will begin to breath again, and as she does, will awaken. She is having Cheyne-Stokes respiration, in which periods of apnea alternate cyclically with periods of hyperpnea. During apnea, this particular patient becomes lethargic and appears to drift off to sleep, while during the hyperpneic phase, she appears more alert.

2. Cheyne-Stokes respiration can occur in a number of clinical settings, but typically occurs in elderly patients with central nervous system disease and heart failure. Autopsy studies have failed to localize a specific site of neurologic damage associated with this abnormal respiratory pattern, and overt cardiac or neurologic disease is not necessarily present. Prolonged circulation time presumably reduces cerebral circulation, while pulmonary congestion produces hypoxemia, increasing the sensitivity of the respiratory control center. Thus, CHF is a classic precipitant of Cheyne-Stokes respiration in elderly stroke patients.

3. The patient's profound neurologic impairment makes expression of symptoms close to impossible. Her lung findings are chronic and are probably not related to acute congestive failure, but to pulmonary scarring or basilar atelectasis. With age, preferential distribution of ventilation to lower lung zones may be impaired during ordinary (tidal volume) breathing. This finding is probably due to age-related loss of pulmonary elastic recoil, which results in a decreased resistance to alveolar collapse. This change is probably further exacerbated by the bed- or chair-bound state. Thus, the finding of rales in such patients is diagnostically useful only if clearly a new finding. On the other hand, a third heart sound is a specific finding in CHF, but is not always audible.

Since the patient is bedridden, examination of the legs is not a reliable method of looking for dependent edema, and the presacral area should be examined. When present, edema of the extremities is a very nonspecific finding in the elderly because of the high prevalence of venous insufficiency. Furthermore, paretic extremities are commonly and chronically edematous in patients without heart failure. This is thought to be due to lack of autonomic supply to the vessels of the extremities. Asymmetric leg edema is also common in elderly heart failure patients without strokes, because venous insufficiency may also be asymmetric.

4. Assuming that this patient has no new neurologic findings, congestive heart failure is a good working diagnosis. An electrocardiogram should be done to rule out myocardial infarction, since this aphasic patient could not complain of chest pain. It is a geriatric "given" that myocardial infarction can present

atypically in the elderly (see Case 30). A chest x-ray should be performed to rule out pneumonia, which can itself be a precipitant of acute cardiac decompensation in the elderly. Since intrusive diagnostic maneuvers are rarely warranted in debilitated patients and since comfort care is of essence, a gentle, clinical approach should be taken. Presumed heart failure should be treated with a thiazide or loop diuretic. If a loop diuretic is chosen, adverse effects can be minimized if the starting dose is low. Furosemide 10 to 20 mg is often effective.

Pearls:

1. Although CHF in the elderly is due to the same spectrum of diseases as in younger adults, underrecognized causes of chronic heart failure in the elderly include senile cardiac amyloidosis and hypertrophic cardiomyopathy. Senile cardiac amyloidosis is present in 50% of people over 60 years of age at autopsy, but is probably clinically significant in only a small minority. This condition is associated with deposition of a form of amyloid (ASc) that is immunologically distinct from amyloid AL and amyloid AA, which are associated with primary and secondary amyloidosis, respectively, and which may also cause cardiac disease in the elderly. Unlike primary and secondary amyloidosis, however, amyloid ASc does not produce disease in other internal organs. None of the three types has been implicated in amyloidosis involving cerebral vessels or other brain structures in Alzheimer's disease.

Hypertrophic cardiomyopathy (HCM), once thought to be a disease of younger adults, is not uncommon in late life. Unfortunately, echocardiographic diagnosis alone may be unreliable, and may be confounded by the autopsy observation that there is an increased septum-to-free-wall ratio in the left ventricle with age. Nonetheless, this condition is probably underdiagnosed in the elderly, due to assumptions that cardiac disease has more common etiologies, due to the presence of other diseases, and due to the fact that it is often morphologically different from young-onset HCM, involving the free wall of the left ventricle. Classic bifid carotid pulse is thought to be absent more often in the elderly, presumably because of underlying age-related stiffness of the arteries. The clinical importance of HCM in the elderly is not known, but the diagnosis should always be kept in mind, since conventional heart failure treatment may be counterproductive.

2. The term "global aphasia" refers to a severe form of nonfluent aphasia, in which language production is virtually absent, although comprehension may be variously retained. Global aphasia is usually due to a lesion involving Broca's area and extending posteriorly, and tends to occur in patients who also have severe hemiplegia.

Pitfalls:

1. The presence of a harsh systolic murmur in a patient with acute CHF raises the suspicion of significant aortic stenosis. Noninvasive evaluation should be considered for prognostic reasons, and aortic valve replacement is a definite option in even very elderly patients who are otherwise robust. However, surgical treatment in debilitated patients such as the present one is rarely considered, since overall quality of life would not be improved.

2. Although Cheyne-Stokes respiration is not commonly associated with pulmonary embolus, this diagnosis should be considered in stroke patients who develop other respiratory difficulties. These patients are at risk because of the tendency for deep venous thrombosis to develop in the paretic limb.

3. Digoxin may provide additional improvement in acute congestive heart failure when added to a regimen consisting of diuretics. However, this renally excreted agent, with its narrow therapeutic-to-toxic ratio, must be used cautiously in the elderly. On the average, an appropriate loading dose in the elderly is no more than 75% of what would be given in a middle-aged patient, and the initial maintenance dose is no more than 50%. Extra caution is advised in patients over 85.

References:

Albert ML, Helm-Estabrooks N. Diagnosis and treatment of aphasia. JAMA 1988;259:1043-1047,1205-1210.

Hodkinson HM, Pomerance A. The clinical significance of senile cardiac amyloidosis: a prospective clinico-pathological study. Q J Med 1977;46:381-387.

Holland J, Milic-Emili J, Macklem PT, Bates DV. Regional distribution of pulmonary ventilation and perfusion in elderly subjects. J Clin Invest 1968;47:81-92.

Kitzman DW, Scholz DG, Hagen PT, Ilstrum DM, Edwards WD. Age-related changes in normal human hearts during the first 10 decades of life. Part II (Maturity): A quantitative anatomic study of 765 specimens from subjects 20 to 99 years old. Mayo Clin Proc 1988;63:137-146.

Plum F, Posner JB. The diagnosis of stupor and coma. Philadelphia: F.A. Davis Company, 1980:35-36.

Pomerance A, Davies MJ. Pathological features of hypertrophic obstructive cardiomyopathy (HOCM) in the elderly. Brit Heart J 1975;37:305-312.

Shenoy MM, Khanna A, Nejat M, Greif E, Friedman S. Hypertrophic cardiomyopathy in the elderly. Arch Intern Med 1986;146:658-661.

Tobin MJ, Snyder JV. Cheyne-Stokes respiration revisited: controversies and implications. Crit Care Med 1984;12:882-887.

Wright JR, Calkins E. Clinical-pathological differentiation of common amyloid syndromes, Medicine 1981;60:429-448.

Gastrointestinal Bleeding

<u>Case 25.</u> A 78-year-old obese woman developed coffee ground vomitus and was admitted to the hospital. She was a nonsmoker and nondrinker and denied the use of aspirin-containing medicines or arthritis pills. Gastroscopy revealed hemorrhagic gastritis.

She recovered quickly with medical therapy. While her subintern was dictating her discharge summary, he saw her waddle up to the nurses' station. Within minutes, he revised his discharge diagnosis.

<u>Clue:</u>

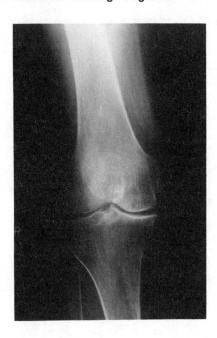

<u>Questions:</u>

1. What risk factor of upper gastrointestinal bleeding should be ruled out?

2. What should be done?

3. What other types of gait disorder are commonly seen in the elderly?

Answers:

1. The patient was observed to have the typical waddling gait of obese women with longstanding painful osteoarthritis (OA) of the knees. This prompted the alert subintern to question the patient further regarding medication intake to rule out gastropathy due to nonsteroidal anti-inflammatory agents (NSAIDs), including aspirin. Although she denied taking offending medication, she had been taking many tablets of Ecotrin (enteric-coated aspirin) and Medipren (ibuprofen) per day, but this information was not elicited until her gait was observed and the right question was asked: "What do you take for pain?" The patient's daughter brought in a bag full of medicines and the etiology unfolded. A friend who suffered from knee pain had recommended Medipren and Ecotrin because they had helped her. The patient did not consider these over-the-counter agents to be medicine at all. "Arthritis pills" are prescribed by doctors, so the patient thought.

When asked how the pills made her feel, she admitted that they gave her a "sour stomach," for which she took Alka-Seltzer, which contains not only antacid but also 325 mg aspirin per tablet. This made her feel worse, so she purchased Alka-Seltzer Extra Strength, which contains 500 mg aspirin per tablet. Then she bled. Although not all formulations of Alka-Seltzer contain aspirin, these and many other over-the-counter agents do, and the trade name usually does not reflect that fact.

In severe OA of the knees, progressive joint space narrowing occurs disproportionately in the medial aspect and often results in genu varum ("bow-leg" deformity), in which the knees are apart although the feet are held together. The deformity, along with compensatory shifting of weight due to pain, alters the center of gravity and impairs balance. The patient compensates by shifting weight from side to side with each step and appears to "waddle." This waddle may mistakenly be attributed to obesity, since patients with severe OA of the knees tend to be obese. This gait pattern occurs in elderly patients without painful joints, and has been referred to as idiopathic "senile gait disorder."

2. The gastritis should be treated with a histamine-2 blocker, such as ranitidine, with sucralfate, which acts by increasing gastric prostaglandin release, or antacid. Gastric prostaglandin, the potent inhibitor of acid secretion and stimulator of mucus secretion in the stomach, is inhibited by NSAIDs. The synthetic prostaglandin E_1 analogue misoprostol (Cytotec) was recently released and is the only agent officially approved for this indication.

In this setting, pains of osteoarthritis can often be adequately treated with less toxic acetaminophen, since many patients have symptomatic relief on doses of aspirin or NSAIDs that are insufficient to produce an anti-inflammatory effect, but sufficient to produce analgesia. If maximum doses of acetaminophen do not help, propoxyphene or acetaminophen plus codeine can be recommended, with the caveat that these agents may produce confusion in the elderly, and codeine is likely to produce constipation.

After the gastric lesion is healed, a nonacetylated salicylate such as salsalate (Disalcid) or choline-magnesium salicylate (Trilisate) may be an option, since they only weakly inhibit PGE2. Other NSAIDs should be avoided unless absolutely necessary, and then should be given only in conjunction with a cytoprotective agent such as sucralfate.

3. Parkinsonian patients have a slow, shuffling gait, accompanied by a paucity of arm movements and a tendency to involuntary acceleration ("festinating gait"). Patients with hemiparesis tend to raise the hip of the affected side and rotate the leg outward, then inward, forming an arc as they take a step. This action compensates for decreased strength of hip and knee flexors and impaired ankle dorsiflexion ("foot drop"). Normal pressure hydrocephalus, an unusual cause of dementia, is associated with gait apraxia in its classic presentation. In gait apraxia, voluntary and sensory pathways are intact, and there is no ataxia, but a central lesion prevents the initiation and completion of the learned function of walking. The classic appearance is that of a "magnetic" gait, in which the legs seem to move heavily. Myelopathy due to vitamin B_{12} deficiency produces sensory ataxia, which manifests as an unsteady gait, and sometimes with a compensatory wide-based gait. Full-blown gait disorder due to pure vitamin-B_{12}-related myelopathy is uncommon nowadays.

Pearls:

1. Heberden's nodes (bony enlargement of the distal interphalangeal joints with narrowing of the joint space) are common findings in the physical examination of elderly patients. Virtually all of the elderly population has radiographic evidence of OA in one or more points while only a minority have pain in the involved joint. Likewise, the presence of Heberden's nodes does not predict disease in other joints.

2. NSAIDs produce gastric more often than duodenal lesions. The variety of pathology, which includes mucosal erythema, erosive or diffuse gastritis, and gastric ulcer, has been termed NSAID gastropathy. The gastric predilection reflects the fact that NSAIDs inhibit the synthesis of protective gastric prostaglandin, while duodenal ulcer is mediated by gastric acid. The risk of NSAID-related gastropathy increases with age, as does the gastric-to-duodenal ulcer ratio in general. This tendency may therefore also reflect the underlying gastric atrophy and achlorhydria that occurs commonly in the elderly.

3. Other gastrointestinal lesions produced by NSAIDs include esophagitis and enterocolitis. Gastritis leads to delayed emptying, transient gastric distension, and reflux. Lesions in the intestine are thought to be related to inhibition of protective prostaglandin secreted by the intestinal cells.

4. The term "osteoarthritis" is used in the United States to designate a condition often termed "osteoarthrosis" in the United Kingdom. It has been argued that the latter term is more descriptive since the condition is associated with bony enlargement of various joints, and clinical inflammation is less common. On the other hand, the initial pathology of OA may involve an inflammatory reaction, resulting in enzymatic destruction of cartilage. Synovial inflammation does, in fact, occur in OA. Primary OA probably is a group of at least two disorders, one genetic and inflammatory involving the hands, the other, involving hips or knees. The latter may be partly mechanical in origin with an inflammatory process that is either primary or secondary.

Pitfalls

1. NSAIDs are very useful and usually well tolerated in the elderly. The increased risk of bleeding is seen primarily in long-term, high dose use. Bleeding is much less common with occasional "PRN" use of these drugs.

2. The presence of Bouchard's nodes in OA, less common than distal Heberden's nodes, should not be mistaken for soft tissue swelling that occurs in rheumatoid arthritis (RA). On the other hand, typical RA does occasionally begin in late life.

3. Other ingredients "hidden" in popular over-the-counter agents that may cause side effects include sympathomimetics, antihistamines, caffeine, alcohol, bismuth, aluminum, sodium, calcium, potassium, and dextromethorphan.

References:

Cunha UV. Differential diagnosis of gait disorders in the elderly. Geriatrics 1988;43(8):33-42.

Lanza FL, Aspinall RL, Swabb EA, et al. Double-blind placebo-controlled endoscopic comparison of the mucosal protective effects of misoprostol versus cimetidine on tolmetin-induced mucosal injury to the stomach and duodenum. Gastroenterol 1988;95:289-294.

Lawrence JS, Bremner JM, Bier F.   Osteo-arthrosis: prevalence in the population and relationship between symptoms and x-ray changes.   Ann Rheum Dis 1966;25:1-24.

Moskowitz RW.   Clinical and laboratory findings in osteoarthritis. In: McCarty DJ.   Arthritis and allied conditions.   Lea & Febiger 1985:1408-1432.

Ravi S, Keat AC, Keat ECB.   Colitis caused by nonsteroidal anti-inflammatory drugs.   Postgrad Med J 1986;62:773-776.

Roth SH, Bennett RE.   Nonsteroidal anti-inflammatory drug gastropathy: recognition and response.   Arch Intern Med 1987;147:2093-2100.

Yazici H, Saville PD, Salvati EA, et al.   Primary osteoarthrosis of the knee or hip: prevalence of Heberden's nodes in relation to age and sex.   JAMA 1975;231:1256-1260.

The Hypochondriac

Case 26. An 86-year-old woman is recovering from a wrist fracture. She has been followed for many years by a physician in the community, but was referred by the hospital orthopedics service to your medical clinic for followup. The patient is a widowed, retired mathematics professor. She lives with her daughter and son-in-law in the suburbs. She has been in good health but has chronic complaints of bloating and belching after meals, constipation, difficulty sleeping, chronic low back pain, and occasional dizziness. A call to her internist reveals that barium studies and blood tests have been normal. He thinks she is "a bit of a hypochondriac," and would not mind if you follow her. Her medications include simethicone 40 mg (Mylicon) for the belching, milk of magnesia for constipation, acetaminophen for back pain, and pentobarbital (Nembutal) for sleep.

On physical exam, the patient is alert and oriented. She is articulate, pleasant, and converses intelligently. Her blood pressure is 140/90 and her pulse is 60 and regular. Her left arm is in a cast. Except for slight kyphosis, her physical examination is normal. The chart reveals that the patient visited the emergency room a few months before because of mild head trauma that gave her a black eye.

On questioning, she reveals that she broke her wrist when she fell at her daughter's home three weeks before. You notice that she has a bruise on her left temple and she says that she fell again and hit her head on the coffee table. When you question her closely about the circumstances surrounding the fall, she says, "Oh, I just fell." You suggest some tests but she wants to get rid of the belching first. You increase the dose of simethicone to 80 mg after meals and urge her to return soon. Thinking that she was a bit evasive concerning the fall, you suspect "elder abuse," and plan to discuss the case with the social worker.

Two weeks later she reports that she has had little relief of her belching. Her physical examination is unchanged. You are willing to consult with a gastroenterologist, but insist that she undertake the tests that you recommend.

Within a week, the cause of the injuries is elucidated and appropriate action is taken. The patient thanks you for your help and promises she will call you after she finds someone to "look into the gastric problem."

Two months later, the patient calls you and says she is "shaking all over." You reassure her and promise to see her early the next week. When she arrives, she says she is still shaking and now is "salivating." You see no evidence of hypersalivation, but notice that her head is bobbing slightly. She has no rigidity of her extremities and her gait is normal. Thinking that this highly educated woman might be concerned that she is developing Parkinson's disease, you explain that she has "essential tremor," which is nothing to worry

139

about. You tell her that if her symptoms are not improved in a week, you will prescribe something.   You have in mind propranolol for the tremor and diphenhydramine (Benadryl) for her complaints of salivation.

A week later, the patient says that the shaking and salivation are getting worse.   Her shoulders and legs are, in fact, shaking quite noticeably. Otherwise she is feeling better--she has not fallen lately and her belching is less noticeable.

Clue:

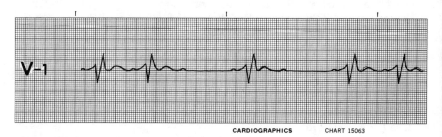

CARDIOGRAPHICS   CHART 15063

Questions:

1. What probably caused the patient's injuries?

2. Of what utility is simethicone in relieving symptoms of belching?   What alternative treatment can be given?

3. What historical information will shed light on the new symptoms of shaking and hypersalivation?

4. Do you think this patient is a hypochondriac?

Answers:

1. Many elderly patients are victims of physical or psychologic abuse that can range from neglect to actual physical violence, but this patient is describing recurrent falls, which require a medical evaluation. Her history is spotty and her review of systems indicated that she suffered from occasional dizziness. Dizziness is a common complaint in the elderly and an actual cause is found only in a minority of cases. In her case, however, the EKG revealed periods of Mobitz type II second degree heart block, which put her at high risk of complete heart block and cardiac syncope. A permanent pacemaker was implanted and the patient did well.

Other causes of recurrent falling in the elderly include perceptual deficits that prevent avoidance of environmental obstacles, transient ischemic episodes, neurologic deficits producing weakness of one or both lower extremities, Parkinson's disease and other causes of gait disorder or postural instability, "drop attacks" and vertebrobasilar insufficiency, orthostatic hypotension, micturition syncope, and any condition or medication that results in problems such as hypotension, dizziness, or weakness.

2. Simethicone is a mixture of silicone polymers that act by changing the surface tension of gas bubbles, causing them to coalesce into larger bubbles that are more easily expelled, or that break. Thus, this agent is thought to relieve symptoms of bloating by dispelling or expelling gas, and seems to work better than placebo. These symptoms may also be due to motility disorders of the gastrointestinal tract. This patient had some degree of gastroparesis, although she was not diabetic, and obtained relief with the dopamine blocking agent, metoclopramide.

Other causes of belching include carbonated beverages, aerophagia produced by chewing gum, anxiety, or wearing badly fitted dentures; attention to these risk factors may cause relief.

3. Like many patients with multisystem disease, this patient has visited more than one physician in a short period of time. Interventions by outside physicians often go unreported. If new symptoms cannot be explained by physical or emotional illness, drug reaction must be considered. Drug history quickly revealed that this patient had visited a gastroenterologist of her own and had received metoclopramide (Reglan), which had markedly reduced her symptoms of belching and bloating. Metoclopramide is a dopamine antagonist, which can produce full-blown, reversible parkinsonism. This patient developed tremor that resembled essential tremor, but may have been an atypical parkinsonian tremor. Hypersalivation in idiopathic Parkinson's disease is thought to be due to dysphagia, which the patient denied; it was therefore attributed to relative cholinergic excess resulting from dopamine depletion. The

symptoms subsided with discontinuation of the medication, but the belching returned. The patient was more annoyed by the belching than the shaking and drooling, and she insisted on resuming the metoclopramide, though she agreed to take a lower dose.

4. Hypochondriasis is the belief that one has a serious illness, based on one's interpretation of physical signs or symptoms, despite the physician's reassurance that no physical illness exists. It is a commonly held view that hypochondriasis is common in old age, but some studies indicate that elderly patients underreport rather than overreport symptoms, a physical explanation for the symptoms being found more often in older than in younger people. The reasons for this underreporting are that illness is often ascribed to "old age," and that patients with dementia are less likely to recognize and report physical ailments. The present patient was found to have a physical problem as the basis for most, if not all, of her complaints (though this is by no means always the case!), and, at least with regard to her bruises, was reluctant to discuss the problem. This may have to do with the psychologic pain experienced by previously robust elderly who start to have falls. When such a person becomes a "faller," he or she starts to feel old, and this sudden reminder of aging can lead to sadness, depression, or denial. Falling can also lead to avoidance of previous activities now viewed as dangerous, and social isolation or inattention to personal affairs may result.

Pearls:

1. When a symptom develops in an elderly patient, it is better to discontinue a drug than to add another one. If the patient's tremor had been treated with propranolol and her hypersalivation with an antihistamine, additional side effects might have occurred. This add-on-a-drug approach is a common way of mismanaging elderly patients.

2. Although it is difficult to know the exact prevalence, an estimated 4% of the American geriatric population suffers from abuse or neglect by a caregiver. This problem occurs in all socioeconomic, racial, and ethnic groups.

Pitfalls:

1. Regular heart rhythm in a falling patient does not rule out potentially dangerous dysrhythmias. Tachy- and bradyarrhythmias can occur paroxysmally, remaining undetected in the office or during monitoring. In addition, troubling dysrhythmias such as atrial tachycardia with block and junctional rhythms produce a normal pulse.

2. Although organic disease must be ruled out, the importance of hypochondriasis among the elderly should not be understated either. Traditionally, hypochondriasis has been thought to be more common in women than in men.

3. Barbiturates are not commonly prescribed as hypnotics nowadays, having been largely supplanted by benzodiazepines. Nonetheless, barbiturates continue to show up in drug regimens of elderly patients. Many patients were prescribed such "out of date" medications in the remote past and continue to take them. No sedative-hypnotic should be stopped abruptly, since severe withdrawal reactions can occur if the medication has been taken more than a few weeks.

References:

Busse EW. Hypochondriasis in the elderly. Compr Ther 1987;13:37-42.

Costa PT, McCrae RR. Somatic complaints in males as a function of age and neuroticism: a longitudinal analysis. J Behav Med 1980;3:245-257.

Indo T, Ando K. Metoclopramide-induced Parkinsonism: clinical characteristics of 10 cases. Arch Neurol 1982;39:494-496.

O'Malley TA, Fulmer TT. Abuse, neglect, and inadequate care. In: Rowe JW, Besdine RW, eds. Geriatric Medicine. 2nd ed. Boston: Little, Brown, 1988:89-98.

O'Malley TA, Everitt DE, O'Malley HC, Campion EW. Identifying and preventing family-mediated abuse and neglect of elderly persons. Ann Intern Med 1983;98:998-1005.

Radebaugh TS, Hadley E, Suzman R, eds. Falls in the elderly: biologic and behavioral aspects. Clin Geriatr Med 1985;1(3).

Stenback A, Kumpulainen, Vauhkonen M. Illness and health behavior in septuagenarians. J Gerontol 1978;33:57-61.

A Diabetic with Poor Vision

Case 27.   A 75-year-old obese diabetic man takes 45 units of NPH plus 12 units Regular insulin daily, and his blood sugar is erratically controlled.   He suffers from no acute illness and does not take medications that impair glucose tolerance.   He had a left cataract extraction quite a few years before, and has an enlarging cataract in the right eye.   He also has a tremor.   Since he is able to understand the principles of insulin administration, you suspect that visual impairments may be to blame.   You suggest cataract extraction, which an ophthalmologist has strongly urged, but the patient says, "The first one didn't work; why should I do it again?"   You suspect that he is not taking his insulin correctly and suggest that his family members assist him, but he shrugs and says, "Oh, they won't do anything."   Dietary counseling has failed to help him lose weight and you insist that he embark on a walking program, but he informs you that   "it's too dangerous for an old man like me to be walking around in that neighborhood."   Your hospital social worker informs you that there are some "serious family problems."

Clue:

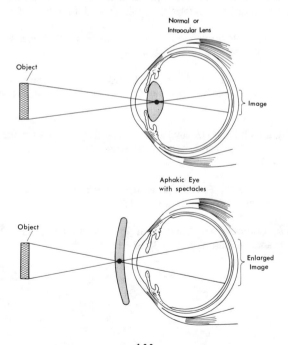

Questions:

1. What approaches can be used to aid him in taking his insulin correctly?

2. What other factors could be contributing to his inadequate diabetic control?

3. Why didn't the first operation "work"? What can be done about this?

4. How does insulin treatment differ in the elderly diabetic?

Answers:

1. In the absence of family assistance (the patient's wife objected to doctors and medical treatment on religious grounds; the son was an irresponsible drug user), the patient's skills and the community's resources need to be maximized. The doctor or nurse should observe the patient draw up and administer his insulin, preferably on a home visit. If he is unable to do this correctly, devices are available to assist those with low vision or impaired manual dexterity. This particular patient tried valiantly to learn to administer his insulin and was observed to be properly using the device that had been given to him. In one out of several observations, however, it was noted that the syringe he felt was drawn up properly was actually filled with air. It was surmised that his impaired vision caused him to fill the syringe although the bottle was near empty. The Visiting Nurse Service then was called upon to prefill syringes once a week.

2. Blood sugar control was still inadequate and he was admitted to the hospital where his blood sugar was controlled on much smaller doses of insulin. The reasons for his poor glycemic control at home were never demonstrated precisely. Dietary indiscretion was probably contributory, and a hypoglycemia-induced counterregulatory reaction (Somogyi effect) was a possibility. Another cause that could not be adequately investigated was the use of the patient's prefilled syringes by his drug-addicted son. This not uncommon form of abuse of the dependent elderly has no ready solution unless a responsible individual can be found to administer the insulin on a daily basis. The present patient had a marginal income, but was not quite poor enough to qualify for Medicaid, which would have paid the high price required for better home care (but see Case 10).

3. The patient's left cataract operation, done quite a few years before, did not include an artificial lens implant, which would have corrected the unilateral aphakia (absence of a lens) and produced near-normal vision. Unilateral cataract excision cannot be corrected with the use of aphakic spectacles, which produce magnification and distortion in the corrected eye (see Clue). Unilateral correction would result in double vision. Contact lenses correct aphakic vision quite well, but are generally too difficult for elderly patients to change on a daily basis, and would be expected to cause this tremulous man a great deal of trouble. An extended-wear lens, changed periodically by a skilled professional, would be useful, if this patient could tolerate one, and if arrangements could be made for regular followup. Extended-wear lenses are poorly tolerated by patients with decreased tear production and those with blepharitis (inflammation of the eyelids), both common problems in the elderly.

The reasons for the patient undergoing unilateral cataract extraction without plans for aphakic correction are worth investigating. Did he fail to tolerate a contact lens? Did he have intraocular disease precluding a lens implant? Were plans made for further surgery that he failed to follow because the first surgery "didn't work"? Answers to these questions will help to ensure a good outcome if further surgery is planned.

One other cause of low vision in patients undergoing cataract extraction is coexistent retinal pathology, such as macular degeneration or proliferative diabetic retinopathy. Elucidation of all eye pathology will determine the outcome and can assist in preoperative counseling. Complications of cataract surgery are uncommon, but include retinal detachment and chronic macular edema, which can impair vision significantly.

This patient should be evaluated for right cataract extraction with intraocular lens implant. A secondary lens implant for the left eye might also be considered. Age is not a limit to cataract surgery; on the contrary, most people undergoing this useful operation are elderly. Moreover, cataract extraction can usually be done under local anesthesia.

4. The same principles apply to the elderly as the younger adult diabetic patient in dosage selection--i.e., dose should be determined by blood sugar. However, "tight" control of blood sugar may not always be desirable, even if achievable. The longterm effects of suboptimal glucose control are not likely to be as important late in life, and hypoglycemia is more likely to result in serious complications such as stroke or myocardial infarction. In addition, the warning signs of hypoglycemia, such as diaphoresis and tachycardia, may be subtle or absent, because of impaired counterregulatory mechanisms. On the other hand, significant hyperglycemia is not desirable; it accelerates the rate of cataract formation, produces dehydration and urinary dysfunction, and may increase susceptibility to bacterial infection.

Pearls:

1. Age alone is associated with complex biochemical changes leading to increased lens opacity. Diabetes can accelerate this process: excess glucose enters the lens where it is enzymatically converted to sorbitol, which is trapped and osmotically draws water into lens fibers. Increased water content alters permeability to other ions, which build up, drawing in more water, until lens fibers swell and rupture. A cataract ultimately can result.

2. Most insulin-requiring elderly diabetics are type II (non-insulin-dependent) diabetics who chronically require insulin because of obesity, or in whom oral hypoglycemic agents are ineffective for reasons that are not well understood. One explanation offered for the failure of oral hypoglycemic agents is that some type II diabetics develop true insulin deficiency over time. Since the oral agents depend for their efficacy on the presence of some insulin, they would not be

expected to work in such patients. However, late-onset diabetes is probably a heterogeneous disorder with more than one pathophysiologic explanation.

3. There is no specific clinical or serologic marker to predict whether insulin-requiring elderly diabetics have type I or type II variety. Nonetheless, it is probably safe to discontinue insulin and give a supervised trial of oral agents to elderly patients who have not previously tried noninsulin treatment. A significant proportion of patients will respond, and will be pleased to discontinue daily injections.

Pitfalls:

1. Aphakic spectacles not only produce a distorted and magnified image, but also fail to provide adequate peripheral vision. Intraocular lens implants offer such an improvement in vision over aphakic spectacles, and are such a practical solution in the elderly, that they are virtually the only treatment considered nowadays, with few exceptions.

2. If regular and NPH insulin are combined in the same syringe, prefilled syringes may lose their preciseness over a period of a few days, since Regular insulin ultimately binds to the protamine-zinc components. Commercially available preparations such as Mixtard can circumvent this difficulty. These products consists of 30% Regular and 70% NPH insulin in a fixed, stable combination, and can be used if this ratio is appropriate for the patient.

3. Although local anesthesia for cataract extraction is far preferable to general anesthesia, the latter should be considered in patients who are deaf, overly anxious, or expected to be agitated, confused, or uncooperative on the operating table.

4. The incidence of complications from intraocular lens implants has decreased dramatically since the early days of this procedure. Nonetheless complications sometimes occur. These include glaucoma, breakage, dislocation, infection, uveitis, and hyphema (hemorrhage into the anterior chamber).

References:

Kilvert A, Fitzgerald MG, Wright AD, Nattrass M. Clinical characteristics and aetiological classification of insulin-dependent diabetes in the elderly. Q J Med 1986;60:865-872.

Liesegang TJ. Cataracts and cataract operations. Mayo Clin Proc 1984;59:556-567,622-632.

Meneilly GS, Greenspan SL, Rowe JW, Minaker KL. Endocrine systems. In: Rowe JW, Besdine RW, eds. Geriatric Medicine. 2nd ed. Boston: Little, Brown, 1988:408-413.

Puxty JAH, Hunter DH, Burr WA. Accuracy of insulin injection in elderly patients. Brit Med J 1983;287:1762.

Acute Hemiparesis

<u>Case 28.</u> An 84-year-old woman is having dinner with her daughter's family when suddenly some food drops out of her mouth. Her son-in-law notices that she is staring into space and asks her what is wrong but she cannot get words out to explain. It appears as though she has dropped her fork and has begun to drool. The family grows alarmed and calls an ambulance, which takes her to the emergency room. Her neurologic symptoms resolve before she reaches the hospital, and she is sent home, having been instructed to take one enteric-coated aspirin daily.

Six months later a similar episode occurs, but this time the symptoms do not resolve.

On physical examination, the patient is alert. Pulse is 72 and irregularly irregular. Blood pressure is 120/60. There is a bruit heard over the left carotid artery. On physical examination there is flattening of the right nasolabial fold. Her right upper and lower extremities are weak.   When asked how she feels, she appears to be attempting an answer but cannot speak. She is unable to cooperate for a full sensory examination but she appears to have slightly decreased sensation to pinprick on the right side. Stool is guaiac negative.

The family tells you that she is being treated for a "heart problem," for which she has been taking medication.

<u>Clue:</u>

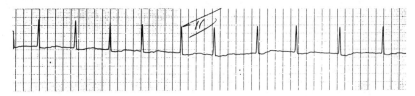

Questions:

1. What is the diagnosis?

2. What is the relationship between the patient's cardiac arrhythmia and the neurologic episode?

3. What is the likelihood that she will have more neurologic problems?

4. What medical treatment is indicated?

5. What preventive measures can be taken?

6. What is "ADL," and what can be done to maximize it in this patient?

Answers:

1.   The patient most likely has had acute cerebrovascular insufficiency involving the left middle cerebral artery.   The exact nature of the insufficiency has yet to be determined.

2.   Although patients with atrial fibrillation (AF) have nearly a six-fold increased risk of stroke than those without AF (and more than ten-fold in the presence of rheumatic valvular disease), it is often difficult to prove a cause-effect relationship in each case.   AF occurs in roughly 5% of community-dwelling and 12% of hospitalized elderly.   Whereas fewer than 10% of middle-aged stroke victims have AF, nearly 40% of stroke patients in this woman's age group do, but cerebrovascular arteriosclerosis is likewise common in the elderly, and age alone is a risk factor for stroke.   It is also difficult to distinguish between thrombosis and embolus on clinical grounds.   Autopsy studies have shown a higher incidence of arterial emboli in stroke patients with AF than those with normal sinus rhythm, but it is not certain if the source of the emboli is in the atrium, since atrial thrombi (also more common in patients with AF) are not always demonstrated.   This patient's stroke was preceded by a transient ischemic episode (TIA) in the same vascular territory, and, on top of that, she has a carotid bruit.   Since classic TIA is not thought to be due to cardiogenic emboli, it is entirely possible that her stroke was due to an embolus from the carotid artery, and that the atrial fibrillation is merely a fellow traveler.

3.   Statistically, there is roughly a 20% risk that this patient will have another stroke within the next year because of the association of AF, whether or not this is an etiologic factor in the present or subsequent neurologic events. The history of TIA itself is associated with a significant risk of stroke within the first year, but a history of TIA confers an equal or greater risk of myocardial infarction, presumably because of the presence of diffuse arteriosclerotic disease.

4.   There is no specific medical treatment for stroke.   However, anticoagulation may reduce the neurologic deficit for "stroke in evolution," and is sometimes used in the management of acute, nonhemorrhagic stroke.   In the setting of AF, such treatment may have more meaning, and anticoagulation is usually recommended in these situations, despite the absence of data from well-controlled studies.

Important treatment consists of ruling out unusual causes of stroke, such as temporal arteritis, and attending to such precipitants of stroke as hypotension or hypoglycemia.   The patient's blood pressure is lower than average for her age.   It would be important to know whether she was being treated for hypertension.   Overtreatment of hypertension may cause a "hypotensive stroke" in elderly patients, by critically reducing perfusion of inadequate cerebral arteries. Gastrointestinal bleeding can also cause a hypotensive stroke, but is unlikely in view of the negative stool guaiac.

An echocardiogram should be considered, since the presence of mural thrombus would probably justify anticoagulation. However, thrombus is seen in an extremely low proportion of cases, even with 2-D echo. This has to do with the imperfect sensitivity of the test, the fact that left atrial thrombi develop in the poorly visualized atrial appendage, and the actual absence in 60 to 83% of embolic stroke cases at autopsy.

Although the need for CT scan in this setting continues to be debated, it has become more or less routine.

5. Prevention of acute complications includes support of the paretic arm to prevent shoulder subluxation, and frequent turning and padding of pressure points to prevent decubitus ulcers.

The science of preventing further neurologic episodes has, unfortunately, not been perfected. Although the source of her presumed embolus is uncertain, aspirin has failed to prevent a stroke. Addition of dipyridamole is unlikely to provide additional protection, even in carotid disease, although there is some disagreement on this point. Longterm oral anticoagulation, keeping the prothrombin time at no more than 1.3 times the control value, should be considered in patients with nonvalvular atrial fibrillation who have had a probable embolic episode, if there is no contraindication, and if the patient is reliable or is in a controlled environment. It may be, of course, that the plaque or thrombus producing the embolus is now dispersed.

6. "ADL" is the expression used to refer to a patient's ability to perform activities of daily living. ADL assessment includes ability to toilet, dress, groom, bathe, ambulate, transfer, and feed. A more sensitive set of functional measures is IADL (instrumental activities of daily living), which include cooking, shopping, handling finances, keeping house, using the telephone, and ability to use transportation. The IADL scale is relevant to community-dwelling elderly, or recovering stroke or fracture patients that are being considered for discharge home, while the ADL scale would perhaps be more relevant for the patient who required institutionalization or around-the-clock home care.

The present patient should undergo physical therapy, in order to maximize physical function; occupational therapy, in order to become able to perform specific tasks; and speech therapy, in order to maximize verbal performance. When neurologic and functional return have leveled off, the patient is said to "plateau." At this point, rehabilitation goals are directed at maintenance of physical and psychologic function.

Pearls:

1. Sometimes the only evidence of past stroke is a residual central seventh (VII) cranial nerve palsy. It is important to distinguish between a "central VII," which involves the corticobulbar pathways, and a "peripheral VII," which is due to damage to the facial nerve itself. Central VII is characterized by weakness of the lower facial muscles and may be manifested as a flattening of the naso-labial fold or crooked smile, and the patient may complain of drooling. Palpebral fissure is occasionally widened, but severe weakness of eyelid closing does not occur. Peripheral VII is characterized by weakness of both upper and lower facial muscles; forehead wrinkles may be decreased on the affected side, and, since the orbicularis oculi muscle is weak, the eye cannot be closed properly and the patient may complain of excessive tearing. The apparent paradox of the central lesion being less severe than the peripheral is due to the fact that crossed fibers from the nondiseased cerebral hemisphere supply the intact lower motor neuron serving the upper part of the face, whereas no amount of cortical input will make the nerve function if the lesion is in the nerve itself.

2. Problems speaking may be due to aphasia or dysarthria. Aphasia (more accurately called "dysphasia" if the deficit is incomplete) implies a problem in the language centers of the brain, which are most often located on the left ("dominant") side of the brain, even in left-handed people. The mechanical apparatus of phonation (tongue, palate, and lips) are intact, but the brain is unable to create normal speech. Writing is generally impaired as well. In dysarthria, there is damage to the neurologic or muscular supply of the organs of phonation; although speech and comprehension are normal, words are slurred and may be unintelligible. Dysarthria is associated with a better general functional outcome than aphasia.

3. Terminology regarding different forms of aphasia is confusing, and there is disagreement among authors. This probably has to do with the complexity of the neurologic structures involved and the overlap of specific language deficits. "Expressive" and "receptive" aphasia are not two distinct entities, but commonly overlap. Nor is an aphasia purely fluent (well articulated speech appearing syntactical while not making complete sense) or nonfluent (sparse production of speech). The classic notions of Broca's and Wernicke's aphasia persist. Broca's aphasia, thought to involve lesions in the territory of the middle cerebral artery, is generally nonfluent, while Wernicke's aphasia, due to a lesion in the posterior superior temporal lobe, is fluent but nonsensical because it is peppered with paraphrasia--i.e., words or parts of them are often substituted for irrelevant words or syllables. While patients with Broca's aphasia often appear extremely frustrated by their inability to speak, those with Wernicke's

aphasia often appear unaware of their deficit, and, since the latter may occur as a result of inferior middle cerebral artery occlusion, significant hemiparesis is often absent. This produces a picture of a functioning individual who fails to understand what is going on. Numerous variations on these traditional distinctions have been described, and the complexity of our understanding of aphasia increases as research tools increase in their sophistication.

Pitfalls:

1. Subluxation of the shoulder is a common complication of acute hemiparesis. A standard preventive maneuver is to put the affected arm in a sling. However, this maneuver may not be without its pitfalls. It is important that the sling be fitted correctly and appropriate measures be taken to prevent spasticity of the paretic arm, or contractures may result.

2. Occasionally, brain tumors are misdiagnosed in the elderly as strokes. The neurologic deficit of a stroke, by definition, is characterized by the suddenness of its onset (although a "stroke in evolution" may develop over a period of hours), while a tumor is characterized by its insidious onset, with focality being a little more vague. This misdiagnosis probably occurs because neurologic deficits in the elderly are often assumed to be cerebrovascular in origin, but a careful history must be obtained.

3. Homonymous hemianopsia is a common deficit that occurs as a result of middle cerebral artery occlusion. Vision is impaired in visual space on the side opposite the lesion (the same side as the hemiparesis). This is a subtle finding, particularly in perceptually impaired patients with left-brain lesions, and can be mistaken for inattention. The stroke patient should be examined carefully for the presence of hemianopsia so that other deficits can be evaluated accurately.

4. The use of aspirin in the prevention of stroke is controversial. Although the antiplatelet effect of low-dose aspirin probably prevents the propagation of small carotid emboli in some people, intramural hemorrhage of the same vessel may occur in others. In the present patient, aspirin simply did not work. A higher dose would not have been any more likely to be effective, and would have increased the likelihood of aspirin-related gastropathy, which is unusual at daily doses of 325 mg. Addition of dipyridamole probably does not enhance protection, but this remains controversial. Platelet inhibitors are not likely to prevent stroke if the source of the embolus is an intracardiac thrombus. In such cases, anticoagulation should be considered.

5. Carotid endarterectomy and other surgical approaches to arteriosclerotic stroke are highly controversial. In general, neurologists and internists feel that

while surgical treatment may prevent recurrence of stroke in the same vascular distribution, it does not reduce overall incidence of stroke recurrence, nor does it reduce 5-year mortality. Patients with carotid artery disease have arteriosclerosis in other arteries, and death most often occurs from myocardial infarction.

References:

Adams RD, Victor M. Principles of neurology. 4th ed. New York: McGraw-Hill, 1989:617-692.

Albert M, Helm-Estabrooks N. Diagnosis and treatment of aphasia. JAMA 1988;259:1043-1047,1205-1210.

Andrews K. Rehabilitation. In: Brocklehurst JC, ed. Textbook of geriatrics and gerontology, 3rd ed. Edinburgh: Churchill Livingstone, 1985:1021-1038.

Branch LG, Meyers AR. Assessing physical function in the elderly. Clin Geriatr Med 1987;3:29-51.

Campbell A, Caird FI, Jackson TFM. Prevalence of abnormalities of electrocardiogram in old people. Brit Heart J 1974;36:1005-1011.

Dunn M, Alexander J, deSilva R, Hildner F. Antithrombotic therapy in atrial fibrillation. Chest 1986;89 (Suppl):68S-74S.

Dyken ML. Carotid endarterectomy studies: a glimmering of science. Stroke 1986;17:355-358.

Geschwind N. Aphasia. N Engl J Med 1971;284:656-658.

Gibson CJ, Caplan BM. Rehabilitation of the patient with stroke. In: Williams TF. Rehabilitation in the Aging. New York: Raven Press, 1984:145-160.

Harrison MJG, Marshall J. Atrial fibrillation, TIAs and completed strokes. Stroke 1984;15:441-442.

Hinton RC, Kistler JP, Fallon JT, Friedlich AL, Fisher CM. Influence of etiology of atrial fibrillation on incidence of systemic embolization. Am J Cardiol 1977;40:509-513.

Hirsh J, Fuster V, Salzman E. Dose antiplatelet agents; the relationship among side effects and antithrombotic effectiveness. Chest 1986; 2 (Suppl):4s-8s.

Jonas S. Anticoagulant therapy in cerebrovascular disease: review and meta-analysis. Stroke 1988;19:1043-1048.

Kannel WB, Abbott RD, Savage DD, McNamara PM. Epidemiologic features of chronic atrial fibrillation. N Engl J Med 1982;306:1018-1022.

Knopman DS, Anderson DC, Asinger RW, Greenland P, Mikell F, Good DC. Indications for echocardiography in patients with ischemic stroke. Neurology 1982;32:1005-1011.

Mitchinson MJ. The hypotensive stroke. Lancet 1980;1:244-246.

Starkey I, Warlow C. The secondary prevention of stroke in patients with atrial fibrillation. Arch Neurol 1986;43:66-68.

Sherman DG, Hart RG, Easton JD. The secondary prevention of stroke in patients with atrial fibrillation. Arch Neurol 1986;43:68-70.

Wolf PA, Abbott RD, Kannel WB. Atrial fibrillation: a major contributor to stroke in the elderly. The Framingham Study. Arch Intern Med 1987;147:1561-1564.

Chronic Hemiparesis

Case 29.   After 6 months of rehabilitation, the patient in Case 28 "plateaus." She has regained some speech but produces few words. Her right arm and leg are very weak.   There is increased tone but no significant spasticity. Impaired plantar flexion in her paretic limb has left her with a "foot drop." She has learned to transfer from chair to bed and toilet, but cannot ambulate without a cane, and sometimes has difficulty standing on her own. She seems to comprehend speech and follows commands regularly. She is able to feed herself if food is prepared, cut, and brought to her. She has difficulty dressing and grooming and requires assistance in handling her personal affairs. She has been living in a skilled nursing facility with a rehabilitation service, and wishes to live in her daughter's home. The family is eager to have her live with them, and is prepared to obtain a home attendant if necessary.

Clues:

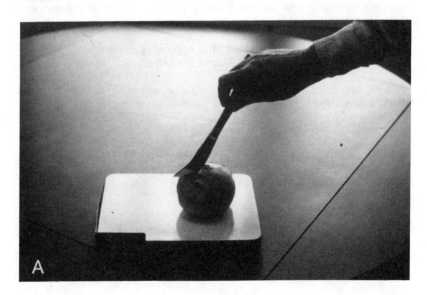

Clues (cont.):

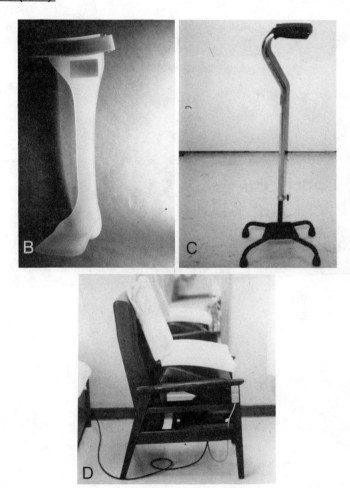

Clues (cont.):

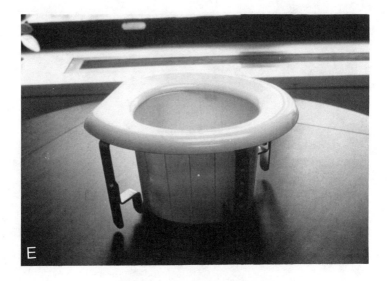

Questions:

1. How can the devices pictured be useful to her?

2. What are some of the late complications and sequelae of stroke, and what can be done about them?

Answers:

1. a. Unique utensils exist so that people with only one useful hand can prepare and eat food. The device pictured here can assist the patient to cut her food on her own. It is being demonstrated on a cutting board that is adherent to the counter and will be of additional help if she wishes to prepare her own food. Numerous other devices are available to assist handicapped people to improve their independence. Velcro closures for shoes and garments, long-handled shoe horns, stocking pulls, and zipper pulls are but a few of the simpler devices that elderly patients are successfully taught to use by the occupational therapist. These devices are not only useful to hemiparetic patients, but those with other musculoskeletal limitations such as Parkinson's disease, arthritis, fractures, and amputations.

b. The posterior leaf splint is lightweight and well tolerated. It is constructed so that it will prevent involuntary plantar flexion and is a very useful "orthotic" in stroke patients whose hemiparesis includes weak dorsiflexion or ankle instability. If there is severe spasticity, this type of orthotic cannot be used. The posterior leaf splint is lightweight and better tolerated than a heavier metal brace.

c. The four-pronged "quad" cane will confer greater stability than an ordinary cane, and is preferred by patients to the more cumbersome and conspicuous walker.

d. Pain, stiffness, or weakness in joints or muscles responsible for extension at the knee and hip make it extremely difficult for people with a variety of disorders to get out of low chairs. Straight-backed arm chairs are the best standard chairs for such patients, but the pictured seat-lift chair gives the patient additional mechanical assistance, and may be particularly useful for a patient with a weak arm.

e. Toilet seats are even lower than standard chairs. The raised toilet seat will be very useful to this patient, and should be installed along with strategically placed arm rails. Independence in toileting is one of the most important parts of rehabilitation. Being put on and off a toilet can be emotionally devastating. Also, since many elderly stroke patients develop unstable bladder and urinary frequency, being able to toilet on one's own can mean the difference between going home or remaining institutionalized.

2. Contractures and pain often occur in paretic extremities. Contractures can be prevented by early institution of range-of-motion exercises, treatment of accompanying pain, and splinting to counteract an imbalance between agonist

and antagonist muscle groups. Antispasticity medications, such as baclofen and diazepam, tend to exacerbate cognitive deficits in elderly patients, and must be used with caution. Chronic pain in paretic extremities can also be due to lesions involving the thalamus, or from mechanical disturbances resulting from spastic or flaccid paralysis of the arm. Mechanical factors include traction or compression neuropathy, shoulder subluxation, or rotator cuff tear from improper moving or positioning of the patient by caregivers. Incorrect or prolonged use of an arm sling may result in adduction and internal rotation contracture and adhesive capsulitis of the shoulder. The "shoulder-hand" syndrome is a painful sequela of hemiplegic stroke. It is an abnormality in the sympathetic nervous system, thought to be a "reflex sympathetic dystrophy" related to mechanical damage to the shoulder. Symptoms consist of progressive pain and decreased range of motion of the affected shoulder, along with swelling and coldness. The pain can be prevented with local steroids or systemic analgesia, accompanied by regular range-of-motion exercises.

Stroke patients are at high risk of falling. The risk is due not only to weakness or spasticity in the leg, but also from visual field deficits, cognitive impairments, and spatial-perceptual deficits. Impaired dorsiflexion with foot drop occurs commonly in hemiparetic patients and can increase the risk of falls by causing tripping.

Immobilized patients are likely to develop decubitus ulcers at pressure points. Sacral decubiti are common in patients who sit all day, especially if they are incontinent. The mainstay in the prevention and treatment of decubitus ulcers is the relief of pressure and avoidance of friction and excessive moisture. Patients who must sit for prolonged periods often benefit from "donut" or "waffle" cushions. The incidence and severity of decubitus ulcers are inversely proportional to nursing time spent.

Poststroke depression occurs in 20 to 60% of patients but may respond well to treatment with supportive therapy, medication, or electroconvulsive therapy. It is commonly unrecognized or treated with a shrug of the shoulder. Dementia in major hemispheric strokes is common, and is most often the result of the stroke itself, although this "vascular dementia" often co-occurs with Alzheimer's disease.

Deep vein thrombosis commonly develops in paralyzed legs and may produce pulmonary emboli. Physicians who specialize in rehabilitation medicine have observed that this is particularly common in patients with left hemiparesis. The explanation for this is that patients with right-sided brain lesions often have spatial neglect of the affected side. They not only bump into objects in that side of space, but fail to move the paretic limb passively. They sometimes lack insight into their deficits, which exacerbates the problem. Since speech is usually unimpaired in patients with right-sided brain lesions, observers and caregivers tend to underestimate the patient's deficits. Spatial neglect is one of many visual-spatial-perceptual problems that occur in these patients.

Urinary incontinence is a common complication of stroke and is discussed in Case 16.

Poststroke seizures occur in 10 to 30% of patients. Although seizures have been reported to occur at the time of onset of the stroke in a minority of cases, it is generally agreed that the usual time of onset is roughly 6 months after the initial stroke. On the other hand, CT studies suggest that seizures may occur as a late sequela of a "silent" stroke. This observation might explain some cases in which stroke appeared to present initially as a seizure. Because only a minority of stroke patients develop seizures, and since these seizures tend to be of the partial motor type, anticonvulsant prophylaxis is generally not given.

Pearls:

1. Normal people shift position automatically, even during sleep, thereby preventing critical increases in capillary pressure that eventually lead to skin breakdown. Paralysis prevents this automatic protective shifting of position, so that stroke patients are at an increased risk of developing decubitus ulcers. This risk increases with age because of age-related skin changes, including thinning of the skin, decreased subcutaneous fat over bony prominences, and sluggish wound healing. The presence of contractures predisposes to decubitus ulcers in unexpected sites.

2. Many patients who require a cane are embarrassed to use one because it makes them "look old," or because they fear that using a cane will make them appear vulnerable and a prey to muggers. For such people, a large umbrella with a heavy rubber tip can be substituted. This confers very good stability and may be more acceptable.

Pitfalls:

1. Although the four-pronged "quad" cane is intended to confer greater stability than an ordinary cane, a patient cannot merely be given this, or any other type of assistive device, without being taught to use it. Poorly taught and cognitively impaired patients may not use ambulatory aids properly, and may fail to rest all four prongs of a quad-cane on the ground, or may hold it backwards and trip over the base. A cane should be held on the side opposite the deficit and planted firmly ahead before moving the impaired limb. Then the first step is taken by the impaired leg and weight planted. Finally the strong leg takes a step. The sequence is: cane, impaired leg, strong leg. The height of the cane

should be adjusted so that the top is at the level of the femoral trochanter and the elbow is flexed 15 degrees.

2. Wheeled walkers are not as stable as standard walkers, but are preferred by many patients because they allow for more speedy ambulation. Patients with instability due to paretic limbs should generally avoid the wheeled walker.

3. Decubitus ulcers are not always what they seem. Occasionally, small ulcers may appear to "blossom" over a short period of time. This occurs if the small ulcer conceals a wider, necrotic crater. Probing or debriding of small ulcers may be required if there is a suspicion that infected tissue lies beneath.

References:

Andrews K. Rehabilitation. In: Brocklehurst JC, ed. Textbook of geriatrics and gerontology, 3rd ed. Edinburgh: Churchill Livingstone, 1985:1021-1038.

Cocito L, Favale E, Reni L. Epileptic seizures in cerebral arterial occlusive disease. Stroke 1982;13:189-195.

Delisa JA, Mikulic MA, Melnick RR, Miller RM. Stroke rehabilitation: Part II. Recovery and complications. Amer Fam Physician 1982;26(6):143-157.

Dupont RM, Cullum CM, Jeste DV. Poststroke depression and psychosis. Psychiatr Clin North Am 1988;11:133-149.

Feigenson JS. Stroke rehabilitation. Outcome studies and guidelines for alternative levels of care. Stroke 1981;12:372-375.

Hier DB, Mondlock J, Caplan LR. Behavioral abnormalities after right hemisphere stroke. Neurology 1983;33:337-344.

Reuler JB, Cooney TG. The pressure sore: pathophysiology and principles of management. Ann Intern Med 1981;94:661-666.

Chest Pain

Case 30. Part 2. An 88-year-old woman complains of "soreness in the chest."
She seems distressed and clutches a bottle of pills in each hand. She asks,
"Should I take this (nitroglycerin)? Should I take this (Valium)? Should I go
out? Should I stay in? What should I do?"

The chest pain is not related to meals or exertion. Neither medication
brings consistent relief. Her physical examination, electrocardiogram, chest x-
ray, and abdominal ultrasound yield no clues. An investigation of the patient's
life stresses is begun.

The patient's husband died 4 years before. She lives alone but has a lot
of friends, and, since her husband's death, has resumed an active social life.
She takes no other medication, except for a multivitamin pill.

Clue:

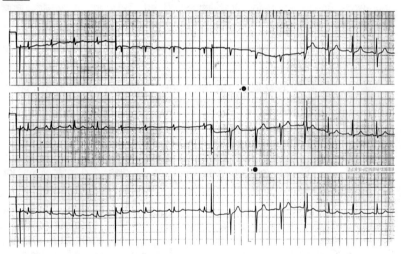

Questions:

1. What information does the patient's EKG contribute to the diagnosis of
ischemic heart disease?

2. How does angina present late in life? Why?

3. What could be troubling an 88-year-old woman?

Answers:

1. Poor R-wave progression on an EKG is suggestive of underlying cardiac disease, but this finding is nonspecific and neither rules in nor rules out cardiac disease. Older patients tend to have a more superior and leftward orientation of the QRS vector than do younger adults. In addition, change in body position appears to affect the precordial leads much more in the elderly than in others, perhaps because of alterations in thoracic anatomy or because of changes in elasticity of the great vessels. Thus, the information available on this patient is quite nonspecific; cardiac pain has neither been ruled in nor out.

2. Angina can present typically, with pain in the chest, jaw, or suprasternal notch, but angina is an uncommon manifestation of cardiac ischemia in people over 85. "Silent" ischemia--or more accurately, "painless" ischemia--occurs more commonly in older patients because the left ventricle tends to stiffen with age. In the ischemic cascade, left ventricular contraction is impaired first, producing characteristic EKG changes, and then pain occurs. If the patient has a stiff ventricle when ischemic heart disease develops, it is likely that symptoms of left ventricular dysfunction will occur early on. Dyspnea or fatigue will cause the patient to rest before pain actually begins. It has also been postulated that pain perception is impaired with age due to alteration in nervous transmission, but the importance of this factor is not known.

3. The patient's frustrated affect suggests that she is suffering some sort of stress, which could be the result of inability to deal with her symptoms, or which could be causing them. Somatic symptoms are a common manifestation of depression and often mask depression in the elderly. Disease itself, and the inability to cope with the involution of health at the end of life, can precipitate depression, but the elderly suffer personal losses as well. Death of a spouse is the most obvious major loss that should be inquired about, but very elderly people often outlive siblings and close friends, and may even outlive their children and grandchildren. It is very important to inquire, specifically, whether a distressed patient has recently experienced the death of any of these important people. This particular patient had functioned well for the 4 years following the death of her husband, to whom she had been married since the age of 18, but had recently started to date again. As a pitfall of her new lifestyle, she had been jilted by a regular gentleman visitor in favor of a younger woman, who herself was over 80 years of age. This information was not volunteered, and was not elicited immediately, perhaps because of the embarrassment that such behavior caused her. She may have viewed dating at her age as unseemly, or may have felt guilt over renewed sexuality.

   This case points up the importance of avoiding age bias when looking into the causes of any symptoms. Sexual feelings are normal in late life, although sexuality has not been well studied in the aged female. Even in the absence of sexual activity, emotional attachments are at least as strong in old age as before. Another overlooked cause of late-onset depression is loss of employment. This factor is especially important in men 60 to 70 years of age, but many people are gainfully employed until extreme old age, and sudden loss of life's work is another problem that should be explored in this setting.

Supportive psychotherapy, reassurance that her distress over the loss of her gentleman friend would pass, and emphasis of the importance of maximizing her social supports were of immense help to this patient. Her chest pain syndrome resolved and she resumed her active social life.

Case 30. Part 2.

Six months later the patient comes in for routine followup. She no longer complains of chest pain. On physical examination, blood pressure is 170/80, pulse is 72 and regular. Lungs are clear. A soft systolic ejection murmur, which has been present for at least 5 years, is heard at the apex. Rectal examination reveals guaiac positive stool.

Colonoscopy is performed and a small malignant tumor is found near the hepatic flexure. Preoperative evaluation begins with an EKG, which is unchanged.

Questions:

1. Should colon surgery be performed on this 88-year-old patient?

2. What are the risks of surgery?

3. What sort of preoperative evaluation should be performed?

4. What peri- and postoperative caveats should be heeded?

Answers:

1.   This patient should be strongly urged to undergo surgery to resect her colon cancer, since early-stage colon cancer is potentially curable with surgical resection, and, since elderly patients who are otherwise well have an operative risk that is nearly as low as younger age groups when surgery is elective. Even if the cancer were found to be invasive, this woman of advanced age could still die of an unrelated cause before the cancer had a chance to metastasize widely.

2.   Perioperative mortality in the elderly is related to the presence of disease, rather than age alone. Very elderly patients who are physically robust do quite well.   Factors that increase peri- and postoperative morbidity and mortality include emergency surgery, congestive heart failure, and poorly controlled hypertension.   Isolated systolic hypertension with systolic pressure less than 200 mm Hg is not an independent risk factor, and aggressive antihypertensive treatment is not called for.

3.   This patient must receive a complete history and physical examination. Laboratory evaluation should be performed to screen for manageable diseases such as diabetes and anemia, and for renal and liver disease, which require specific perioperative precautions. Her chest pain syndrome was probably not cardiac in origin, but even if it had been, stable angina is not an independent risk factor for surgery, and exercise stress testing is not routinely warranted. In any case, many elderly have baseline ST-T wave abnormalities and musculoskeletal problems, limiting the interpretation of stress testing. Myocardial infarction in the previous 6 months increases the risk of perioperative cardiac morbidity and mortality, but her EKG has remained unchanged for 6 months, if not longer.

4.   As with other groups of drugs, general anesthetic agents exhibit pharmacokinetic and pharmacodynamic changes in the elderly, requiring dose adjustments.   Induction of anesthesia may be hastened, and recovery from anesthesia and paralytic agents may be prolonged. Prolonged recovery leads to postoperative confusion and an increased incidence of decubitus ulcers and pneumonia. Baroreceptor responses to anesthesia may be dampened so that hypotension may not produce adequate reflex tachycardia, leading to intraoperative cardio- or cerebrovascular complications. Impaired cough reflex and loss of elastic recoil with inappropriate small airway closure are among the pulmonary changes that may increase the susceptibility to pneumonia, and weaning from the respirator may be prolonged.

Deep vein thrombosis is a common postoperative problem in the elderly, and subcutaneous "miniheparin" is often warranted, although it may be ineffective in patients undergoing orthopedic procedures. Postoperative cardiac arrhythmias are common because of underlying cardiac disease, but respond well to treatment.

Pearls:

1. The incidence of colon cancer increases dramatically with age. The biologic nature of this malignancy does not seem to change with age, but age-corrected survival rates for surgically treated colon cancer are better for the elderly, when calculated on an actuarial basis, than they are for the young.

2. The incidence of benign colonic adenomas also increases with age, so that as many as 60% of elderly are found to have adenomas at autopsy. These lesions are felt to have malignant potential and should be excised, although it is not known what proportion of them, left alone, will develop into carcinomas.

Pitfalls:

1. Digoxin is commonly given empirically at the time of surgery as prophylaxis against congestive heart failure (CHF), or to treat perioperative CHF. Perioperative CHF is often due to intraoperative fluid overload, and should not commit the patient to longterm treatment.

2. Low-lying rectal cancer is a more difficult management problem in the elderly, requiring the more complicated abdominoperineal resection and necessitating permanent colostomy. Surgical morbidity and mortality are higher with this type of surgery than simpler anterior approaches required for cancers found higher up in the colon, and require careful preoperative evaluation and strict individualization in terms of decisions to operate.

3. Ferrous iron preparations have been reported to cause false positive stool guaiac tests. These reports have been criticized as being based on subjective criteria in a situation where dark stool color precludes a true, double-blind test. However, the reports are credible and it is probably prudent to avoid iron preparations for a few days prior to collecting the stool. This patient was, in fact, taking a vitamin preparation and the constituents should have been noted, although the amount of iron in multivitamins is much smaller than that used in the studies of false positivity. On the other hand, ascorbic acid (vitamin C) at doses of more than 500 mg per day, a dose found in many popular vitamin preparations, is not completely absorbed by the gastrointestinal tract so that much of the dose appears in the stool. Since ascorbic acid inhibits the pseudoperoxidase activity of heme, upon which the guaiac test reactivity depends, moderate and high doses of vitamin C can cause a false <u>negative</u>

reaction. Other factors that may produce false positive stool guaiac include bismuth, and meat and some other dietary constituents.

4. Anticoagulation may be highly effective in preventing postoperative DVT, but is generally ineffective in hip fracture patients. This is because the fracture triggers the coagulation cascade and thigh vein thrombosis is often present even before surgery occurs.

References:

Boghosian SG, Mooradian AD. Usefulness of routine preoperative chest roentgenograms in elderly patients. J Am Geriatr Soc 1987;35:142-146.

Brandt LJ. Gastrointestinal disorders of the elderly. New York: Raven Press, 1984:324-355.

Cohn PF. Silent myocardial ischemia. Ann Intern Med 1988;109:312-317.

Flugelman MY, Halon DA, Shefer A, Schneeweiss A, Peer M, Dagan T, et al. Persistent painless ST-segment depression after exercise testing and the effect of age. Clin Cardiol 1988;11:365-369.

Gerson MC, Hurst JM, Hertzberg VS, Doogan PA, Cochran MB, Lim S, et al. Cardiac prognosis in noncardiac geriatric surgery. Ann Intern Med 1985;103:832-837.

Gerstenblith G. Noninvasive assessment of cardiac function in the elderly. In: Weisfeldt ML. The aging heart. New York: Raven Press, 1980:247-267.

Gibson JR, Mendenhall MK, Axel NJ. Geriatric anesthesia: minimizing the risk. Clin Geriatr Med 1985;1:313-321.

Goldman L, Caldera DL, Nussbaum SR, Southwick FS, Krogstad D, Murray B, et al. Multifactorial index of cardiac risk in noncardiac surgical procedures. N Engl J Med 1977;297:845-850.

Johnson JC. Perioperative care in cancer surgery. Clin Geriatr Med 1987;3:463-471.

Lifton LJ, Kreiser J. False-positive stool occult blood tests caused by iron preparations. Gastroenterology 1982;83:860-863.

Mohr DN. Estimation of surgical risk in the elderly: a correlative review. J Am Geriatr Soc 1983;31:99-102.

Murphy E. Social origins of depression in old age. Br J Psychiatr 1982;141:135-142.

Olbrich O, Woodford-Williams E. The effect of change of body position on the precordial electrocardiogram in young and aged subjects. J Gerontol 1953;8:56-62.

Ruegg RG, Zisook S, Swerdlow NR. Depression in the aged, an overview. Psychiatr Clin North Am 1988;11:83-99.

Snyder SK. Surgical treatment of low-lying carcinoma of the rectum. Clin Geriatr Med 1985;1:485-492.

Thienhaus OJ. Practical overview of sexual function and advancing age. Geriatrics 1988;43:63-67.

High Intraocular Pressure

<u>Case 31.</u>   An 80-year-old woman is being treated for chronic open angle glaucoma and hypertension. Her medications include hydrochlorothiazide 25 mg daily, prescribed by you, and timolol (Timoptic) 0.5% 2 drops in both eyes twice daily, prescribed by her ophthalmologist.

The patient is in your office for a routine blood pressure check. She has a "bad cold," but doesn't want any medication for it "on account of the glaucoma." She expresses worry over the fact that her intraocular pressure is difficult to control, which prompted her ophthalmologist to prescribe a new medication, a "big white pill." She intimates that she has a friend who "went blind" from glaucoma, and she feels that her own vision is getting worse--she has been having trouble reading signs and has been having some trouble reading fine print for awhile. She also says that she heard on the radio that eye drops can cause serious side effects, but is reluctant to discuss this with her eye doctor because "he is always so busy."

The patient's blood pressure is 160/90.

<u>Clue:</u>

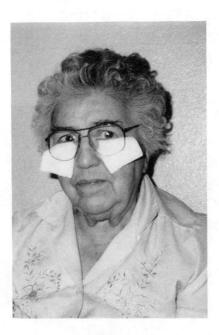

Questions:

1. What systemic effects can be produced by glaucoma drops? How does this happen?

2. What factors could be interfering with control of her intraocular pressure (IOP)?

3. What is the "big white pill" and what should be done about it?

4. What could be causing the patient's visual difficulties?

Answers:

1. Timolol (Timoptic) is one of several ophthalmic agents with beta-adrenergic blocking activity. Ophthalmic agents can be readily absorbed systemically during ophthalmic administration. They may enter the nasolacrimal duct through the puncta of the eye and thereby gain access to the nasal mucosa where they are easily absorbed. Drug that is not absorbed there reaches the nasopharynx and can be swallowed. Vessels of the conjunctivae and other nearby structures account for some systemic absorption. Direct absorption of beta blockers into systemic circulation avoids "first-pass" hepatic metabolism, and increases the systemic potency of these agents, so that even though small amounts are absorbed, typical symptoms of beta blockade may result, including bradycardia, brochospasm, and hypotension. Depression, confusion, and exacerbation of myaesthenia gravis have also been reported with ophthalmic beta blockers. Ophthalmic agents may also participate in systemic drug-drug interactions.

Other topical agents used for glaucoma, such as epinephrine, and the parasympathomimetic agent pilocarpine, produce systemic effects as well. Epinephrine may cause hypertension and arrhythmias, while pilocarpine may precipitate asthma, diarrhea, and hypersalivation. Systemic absorption can be reduced if the punctum is occluded during instillation and for at least 15 seconds afterwards. Also, if the patient is able to tilt the head to the ipsilateral shoulder, excess medication can run out of the eye across the lateral canthus.

2. Instillation of eye drops may be difficult for elderly people because impaired manual dexterity may make it difficult to squeeze small dispensers, and impaired range of motion of the neck may prevent proper positioning of the head. Diminished upward gaze, a normal aging phenomenon, further compounds the problem. This particular patient, however, has ectropion, an eversion of the lower lids that is caused by age-related skin laxity. This condition is causing her eye drops to literally fall out of her eyes, which was not noted until her physician found her in the waiting room with gauze anchored under her glasses. In other situations, ectropion may increase the reservoir area for the drops and may lead to increased systemic absorption of drug. This patient should be instructed to close each eye for at least 15 seconds after instillation, with the puncta occluded, so that the ophthalmic solution is delivered to the site of action.

Fear of side effects could be reducing her compliance, and reassurance is called for.

3. The large, white pill is acetazolamide (Diamox), a carbonic anhydrase inhibitor that reduces the formation of aqueous humor, presumably by altering ion transport associated with the secretion of aqueous humor. This agent is

known for its propensity to produce metabolic acidosis, but, when given in conjunction with thiazide diuretics, may produce severe hypokalemia. As exemplified in this case, elderly patients often go to more than one doctor, and may receive conflicting prescriptions if a careful drug history is not taken by each physician. Measurement of serum electrolytes is a necessity. Her potassium level, previously normal, was 2.7 mEq/L. As a practical solution, hydrochlorothiazide was discontinued by her primary care physician and potassium repleted. Blood pressure remained under control.

Acetazolamide may also produce numbness and tingling sensations in the extremities, lethargy, and reduced appetite, symptoms that often reduce the patient's compliance with the drug regimen.

4.   Uncontrolled open angle glaucoma tends to produce insidious loss of peripheral vision, so when central field symptoms are described, coexisting problems may be at fault. A common cause of central visual loss in the nondiabetic elderly is macular degeneration. Cataracts can cause or exaggerate visual field defects that are often confused with glaucomatous changes, but that may resolve with cataract excision. Visual acuity may also be impaired by pilocarpine drops, still used widely for glaucoma. Pilocarpine is a miotic and produces a pinpoint pupil. If a cataract is also present, light is focused through its center and a very blurred image is produced.

Pearls:

1.   Epidemiologically, glaucoma is associated with systolic arterial hypertension. The reasons for this association are unclear but it has been theorized that arterial hypertension leads to small vessel disease, which reduces flow to the optic nerve or disrupts filtration of aqueous humor. Overtreatment of systemic hypertension could theoretically worsen glaucoma by reducing perfusion pressure of the optic nerve head. This interesting association has not been well studied.

2.   There is no absolute definition of high intraocular pressure. A working definition sets the cutoff at 21 mm Hg, the pressure above which a patient is said to have "intraocular hypertension." If there is evidence of optic nerve damage or glaucomatous visual field deficit, the patient is defined as having glaucoma, but a form of glaucoma ("low tension glaucoma") exists in which glaucomatous deficits occur despite pressures below 21, often in the low teens. Low tension glaucoma is thought to be due to impaired vascularity of the optic nerve head with a resultant imbalance between IOP and perfusion pressure of the nerve head. In these cases, IOP must be lowered still further to prevent additional optic nerve damage and visual loss.

3. Topical beta blockers have supplanted pilocarpine in popularity for the treatment of open angle glaucoma. They are highly effective, increase compliance because they need be given only twice a day, and do not produce miosis, which in itself can impair vision. Pilocarpine and other agents are often used for adjunctive treatment if IOP is not controlled, or if the patient cannot tolerate beta blockers.

Pitfalls:

1. Agents with a tendency to cause mydriasis, such as topical or systemic anticholinergic or adrenergic agents, may precipitate an attack of acute angle closure glaucoma, so that "cold tablets" and a variety of other medications are contraindicated in patients with that condition. However, at least 95% of elderly glaucoma patients have chronic open angle glaucoma, which is not adversely affected by these medications. Although this patient will survive without a cold tablet (and will probably be too anxious to take one anyway), useful medications such as antihistamines, antidepressants, and certain hypertensives will not worsen intraocular pressure in open angle patients, and need not be withheld for that reason.

2. Systemic, but particularly topical ophthalmic steroids can raise intraocular pressure in a small proportion of the general population, while patients with open angle glaucoma or a family history of the disease are unusually sensitive to this effect. Steroids interfere with aqueous humor dynamics by complex, imperfectly understood mechanisms, and should be used with extreme caution in at-risk individuals, if at all.

References:

Carel RS, Korczyn AD, Rock M. Association between ocular pressure and certain health parameters. Ophthalmol 1984;91:311-314.

Epstein DL, Grant WM. Carbonic anhydrase inhibitor side effects. Arch Ophthalmol 1977;95:1378-1382.

Leske MC. The epidemiology of open-angle glaucoma: a review. Am J Epidemiol 1983;118:166-191.

Selvin BL. Systemic effects of topical ophthalmic medications. S Med J 1983;76:349-358.

Shields MB. Textbook of Glaucoma. Baltimore: Williams & Wilkins, 1987.

Five Patients in Need of Antibiotics

Case 32.

A. A 90-year-old man is transferred from the nursing home to an acute care hospital because of fever, neutrophilia, and altered mental status. He has an indwelling urethral (Foley) catheter in place. A "routine" culture 1 week ago revealed greater than 10^5 colonies of Proteus species sensitive to ampicillin.

B. An 83-year-old smoker is brought to the emergency room by his wife because of cough and lethargy. Physical examination reveals decreased breath sounds. Chest x-ray demonstrates hyperinflated lungs, depressed diaphragms, and no infiltrate. Purulent sputum is found on the pillow case of his stretcher. He received pneumococcal vaccine several years before.

C. A 92-year-old woman with end-stage Alzheimer's disease develops fever and lethargy. She resides in a nursing home, and is fed through a nasogastric tube. There is a "stage 2" decubitus ulcer on her sacrum and "stage 1" changes on her left ischial tuberosity. Urine obtained by straight catheter is normal.

D. A 79-year-old community-residing man with chronic venous stasis and edema develops cellulitis. He does not have diabetes.

E. An 82-year-old woman with terrible teeth requires extensive dental work. She has a history of osteoarthritis and has undergone total hip replacement.

Questions:

1. Suggest a likely source of infection or type of bacterial organism responsible for the conditions in patients A through D. What should be your approach to treatment of the infection?

2. Do you think the dentist should be informed about patient E's hip prosthesis? Why?

3. In what clinical circumstances is "empiric treatment" justified?

Answers:

1. A. Although this patient must be examined for other sites of infection, particularly the respiratory tract, the bladder is the most obvious source. Spinal tap is indicated in these cases, but is usually negative. Altered mental status is extremely common in debilitated elderly with systemic infections, even when the infection is outside the central nervous system.

It should not be assumed that a systemic infection in this case is due to Proteus species, since bladders that contain indwelling catheters are usually colonized with several organisms. Different organisms will grow out on different days, making "routine" cultures unjustified. Blood cultures should be done, and the patient should be treated with broad spectrum antibiotics covering gram-negative enteric organisms, unless a gram stain of the urine instructs otherwise: not uncommonly, urinary tract infections are due to enterococcus or other gram-positive cocci, which, of course, must be treated by an entirely different set of antibiotics.

B. The answer is likely to be found if the tell-tale sputum is smeared on a slide and a gram stain is prepared. This patient probably has emphysema and his smear should be examined closely for the presence of small pleomorphic gram negative rods (hemophilus influenza), which are often not seen at first glance, but frequently cause pneumonia in emphysema patients. In this case, the smear revealed many polymorphonuclear leukocytes and gram-positive diplococci. The negative chest x-ray does not rule out pneumonia, since pulmonary infiltrates are frequently radiographically inapparent in the presence of hyperinflation.

If the patient had not produced this diagnostic sputum, one would also have to consider the possibility of Legionnaires' disease. This is a relatively uncommon cause of pneumonia, but age and cigarette smoking are risk factors for sporadically occurring disease.

The history of pneumococcal vaccination does not preclude the diagnosis of pneumoccal pneumonia, since the strain infecting him may not have been present in the vaccine that he received. Moreover, if he was vaccinated several years ago, he might have received a 14-valent preparation, which was in use prior to institution of the 23-valent preparation currently in use. Finally, many chronically ill elderly do not mount a sufficient antibody response to pneumococcal vaccine to guarantee immunity. Assuming that no other site of infection exists, this patient should be treated for pneumococcal pneumonia.

C. Lethargy is a nonspecific symptom in the presence of infection, and requires a thorough physical evaluation and appropriate cultures. The skin of a bedridden, mute patient must be carefully examined for the presence of decubitus or vascular ulcers. Infected teeth are other underrecognized sources of systemic infection in the elderly.   Even nondemented elderly may have extensive dental caries with little or no pain.   Mild viral infections and simple dehydration may also produce fever and lethargy in elderly patients, particularly if they are debilitated.

This patient's decubitus ulcers are most likely not a cause of her new problem.   Stage 1 lesions are not really ulcers, but consist of epidermal erythema, swelling, and heat, and resolve when pressure is removed for 24 hours.   Stage 2 ulcers penetrate to the dermis, but, according to a commonly used classification, do not involve subcutaneous fat.   Stage 1 lesions are treated by removal of pressure and moisture, and avoidance of friction, while stage 2 lesions should, in addition, be cleaned, debrided, and dressed with gauze or hydrocolloid dressings (see Case 19).   Stage 3 ulcers penetrate fat, while stage 4 ulcers involve muscle or bone, and are far more likely than superficial ulcers to produce systemic infection requiring systemic antimicrobial therapy.   Topical antibiotic treatment has limited usefulness, since decubitus ulcers exist in a polymicrobial environment and are easily contaminated by skin, enteric, and environmental bacteria.

This patient is at high risk of developing aspiration pneumonia.   Contrary to the belief of some practitioners, who insert nasogastric tubes in order to reduce the risk of aspiration, large- and small-bore nasogastric tubes actually increase the risk by impairing swallowing of saliva and by reducing lower esophageal sphincter pressure, increasing reflux.   Neurologically impaired elderly, furthermore, often have an impaired cough reflex and swallowing difficulties.

The oropharynx of elderly people is often colonized with gram-negative organisms, whether they have teeth or not.   The likelihood of gram-negative colonization is increased in institutionalized patients, many of whom are prone to the development of aspiration pneumonia.   Although studies have not attempted to correlate specific mouth organisms with etiologic agents in pneumonia, aspiration pneumonia in nursing home patients is typically due to a mixture of anaerobes and aerobic gram-negative organisms.   This patient is very likely to have aspiration pneumonia, but pneumoccal pneumonia is also common in nursing home patients, and should be considered when selecting antibiotics.

D.   Cellulitis in nondiabetic elderly is usually due to staphylococcal or streptococcal organisms.   Since cultures obtained by needle aspiration or punch biopsy are positive in fewer than 25% of specimens, and blood cultures even less sensitive, this conclusion is largely derived from the good response derived by patients from antibiotics such as nafcillin, penicillin, and erythromycin.   Diabetic patients are more likely to have cellulitis due to gram-negative organisms, and occasionally develop fulminant infection with gas-producing Clostridium species.

2. Heart valves are not the only prostheses that can become infected as the result of bacteremia. The total joint arthroplasty is particularly vulnerable and may become infected when seeded by bacteria from infection elsewhere. The actual risk of joint infection from dental procedures, however, is not known, and it has been argued that the risk is slight. Most late infections of prosthetic joints are due to Staphylococcus aureus, beta hemolytic streptococcus, and occasionally, gram-negative organisms, while endocarditis related to dental procedures is most commonly caused by viridans streptococci, and occasionally to S. aureus. Despite the skepticism surrounding the relationship of dental procedures to late infection, over 90% of orthopedists recommend antibiotic prophylaxis with cephalosporins. If this reasoning is to be applied, it should be extended to patients undergoing urologic or intestinal procedures as well.

There is even less unanimity regarding antibiotic prophylaxis for patients with partial prostheses inserted for hip fractures, which can become infected by bacterial seeding from distant infection.

3. Empiric treatment is justified in the presence of an infectious disease emergency, such as impending septic shock, altered mental status, or suspected pneumonia, which can develop into a medical catastrophe rather abruptly in elderly patients. Patient discomfort often demands empiric treatment, notably in acute urinary tract infection, and some upper respiratory infections. Empiric treatment is commonly given in nursing homes, where laboratory support is not always readily available, or where aggressive attempts to obtain cultures may be deemed inappropriate in seriously debilitated patients. Empiric treatment is warranted in conditions such as cellulitis, where microbiologic confirmation is difficult, and frequently warranted when the source of infection is a site prone to polymicrobial colonization, such as deep decubitus ulcers, the chronically catheterized bladder, or aspiration pneumonia.

An attempt should always be made to obtain specimen for culture, and it is imperative that smears be made for appropriate stains, and evaluated as soon as possible. This is particularly important in the setting of pneumonia, which is often caused by anaerobic organisms or pneumococcus. Anaerobes can only be cultured if the specimen is obtained by closed methods, such as the invasive and potentially dangerous transtracheal aspiration, which is rarely justified in chronically debilitated patients. Pneumococcus and certain other aerobic organisms do not grow out readily in routine culture media. The absence of organisms on a sputum gram stain, despite the presence of abundant inflammatory cells, raises the suspicion of Legionnaires' disease or tuberculosis. Mycoplasma pneumonia is rare in the elderly.

Pearl:

Chronic antibiotic therapy does not reduce the incidence of urinary tract infection in longterm catheterized patients. Rather, chronic suppression merely promotes the growth of resistant strains. Within a week of catheter insertion, infection rate approaches 100%. The only definitive treatment is removal of the catheter. If the patient does not have significant urinary retention, removal of the catheter is almost always justified.

Pitfalls:

1. Chronically ill, debilitated elderly (cases A and C) are often colonized with organisms in more than one location. When presentation is nonspecific, the most common sites of infection are the urinary tract and the respiratory tract. It is often necessary to "cover for both," until clinical or microbiologic information dictates otherwise.

2. Ethical considerations must be taken into consideration when decisions are being made about whether to give antibiotics to severely debilitated, hopelessly ill patients. Enteral administration of antibiotics is noninvasive and can be considered part of "comfort care," but may be withheld if it is in accordance with a patient's expressed or previously expressed wishes. Comfort care may include keeping patients out of an acute care setting, which is geared to swift, aggressive, and often, invasive treatment. Withholding antibiotics is associated with high mortality in nursing home patients, so that a decision to withhold a medically indicated antibiotic should be made only after close, informed discussion with patient, family members, or other trusted caregivers. Nursing and other staff should also enter into these discussions when appropriate.

References:

Bentley DW, Torkelson A. Pneumonia in the institutionalized elderly. Gerontologist 1980;20 (pt 2): 66 (abstract).

Breitenbucher RB. Bacterial changes in the urine samples of patients with long-term indwelling catheters. Arch Intern Med 1984;144:1585-1588.

Brown NK, Thompson DJ. Nontreatment of fever in extended-care facilities. N Engl J Med 1979;300:1246-1250.

Ciocon JO, Silverstone FA, Graver M, Foley CJ. Tube feedings in elderly patients. Indications, benefits, and complications. Arch Intern Med 1988;148:429-433.

England AC, Fraser DW, Plikaytis BD, Tsai TF, Storch G, Broome CV. Sporadic legionellosis in the United States: the first thousand cases. Ann Intern Med 1981;94:164-170.

Health and Policy Committee. American College of Physicians. Pneumococcal vaccine. Ann Intern Med 1986;104:118-120.

Jaspers MT, Little JW. Prophylactic antibiotic coverage in patients with total arthroplasty: current practice. J Am Dent Assoc 1985;111:943-948.

Lutomski DM, Trott AT, Runyon JM, Miyagawa CI, Staneck JL, Rivert JO. Microbiology of adult cellulitis. J Fam Practice 1988;26:45-48.

Micolle LE, McLeod J, McIntyre M, MacDonell JA. Significance of pharyngeal colonization with aerobic gram-negative bacilli in elderly institutionalized men. Age Ageing 1986;15:47-52.

Norden CW. Prevention of bone and joint infections. Am J Med 1985;78(6B):229-232.

Reuler JB, Cooney TG. The pressure sore: pathophysiology and principles of management. Ann Intern Med 1981;94:661-666.

Seiler WO, Stahelin HB. Practical management of catheter-associated UTIs. Geriatrics 1988;43(8):43-48.

Simberkoff MS, Cross AP, Al-Ibrahim M, Baltch AL, Geiseler PJ, Nadler J, et al. Efficacy of pneumococcal vaccine in high-risk patients: results of a Veterans Administration cooperative study. N Engl J Med 1986;315:318-327.

Valenti WM, Trudell RG, Bentley DW. Factors predisposing to oropharyngeal colonization with gram-negative bacilli in the aged. N Engl J Med 1978;298:1108-1111.

A Centenarian

Case 33.   An elderly black woman comes to the emergency room of a large teaching hospital because of weakness. She is found to have atrial fibrillation with a rate of 38 beats per minute.

On physical examination, she is alert and oriented. She is in no acute distress and tells the admitting resident that she feels a little weak, but has experienced no other symptoms recently. Blood pressure is 148/90. In the left breast, there is a movable, rock-hard mass measuring 10x10 cm in diameter. There is no ulceration or erythema. She has no hepatomegaly or jaundice. There is a palpable lymph node less than 1 cm in diameter in the left axilla. Neurologic examination is normal.

Her clinic chart is retrieved and reviewed. At age 93 she developed a mass in her right breast but was thought to be too old for surgery. Two years later her presumed breast cancer was treated with hormones and radiation therapy. At age 97 she developed a lump in her left breast. Aspiration biopsy revealed "carcinoma, small cell type," but she and her physicians felt that she was too old for treatment.   She did well and continued to visit the clinic, where she was treated for chronic atrial fibrillation with digoxin. Digoxin had recently been discontinued because of occasional pulse rates under 60.

She thinks it is quite remarkable that she has lived so long, she says, smiling slightly, and sighing.

The patient is a widow, who lives alone and cares for herself. She is active in her church and has a lot of friends.   Her picture was recently in the newspaper on the occasion of her 102nd birthday.

Cardiology consult is called, and it is decided that, "because of the patient's age, advanced cancer, and asymptomatic bradycardia," a pacemaker should not be inserted. She is admitted to the hospital's intermediate care unit for "disposition."

Questions:

1. How would you have handled this case?

2. What might she be sighing about?

3. What do you think happened?

4. What might have happened?

5. How does the life expectancy of a black American woman differ from her white counterpart?

Answers:

1. I hope you would have at least <u>considered</u> putting in a pacemaker. Her nonspecific symptom of weakness could certainly have been attributed to bradycardia, which was of recent onset. The fact that she came to the emergency room was also something new, requiring close attention. A pacemaker is not a ridiculous suggestion at the age of 102. This patient was remarkably youthful for her chronologic age, and was entitled to be taken seriously.

2. She may well be thinking that her "time has come." Elderly people who have been doing "remarkably well" recognize, nonetheless, that death may not be far away. A hospitalization may be viewed as "the end." Patients may either resist hospitalization for this reason, or accept it all too readily. This particular woman, who was religious, was quite prepared to meet her maker, and accepted the decision not to treat without argument. Thus, when the intermediate care unit was invaded by angry geriatricians, ready to go to war with the cardiologists, they found a placid woman, who, along with her pastor, did not join in on the excitement.

3. This patient had a stroke, while the argument raged between the physicians. She died a few weeks after that.

4. If a pacemaker had been inserted, and if this had prevented the stroke, she might have had some more useful life. Just how much longer is uncertain. The presence of atrial fibrillation itself increases stroke risk in the elderly.

One can argue that she might have suffered eventually from the effects of metastatic cancer, but the biologic nature of her tumor appeared to be quite indolent. After 9 years, she has gone beyond the average survival for treated breast cancer patients over 80, and might have done quite well on tamoxifen, which was not available in the early days of her tumor, and which is very well tolerated.

There is little information about breast cancer in centenarians. Autopsy studies have shown an increased incidence, with age, of malignant tumors undetected during life; these tumors, furthermore, tend to be nonmetastatic. This phenomenon has been noted particularly in people over the age of 85, and has been described for prostate, lung, colon, breast, and kidney malignancies. Several studies have hinted at a decreased death rate from certain cancers among the very old, although this probably is related in part to the increased death rate from heart disease and strokes, or the fact that people with more indolent tumors are the ones who survive longer. A biologic explanation for this peculiarity is that tumor growth requires immunologic help and that tumor-enhancing mechanisms involving T-lymphocytes are less active with age. This is one expression of age-related T-cell immunosenescence (see Problem 16, Part II), but in this case, a beneficial one. Biologic sluggishness of geriatric neoplasms continues to be an intriguing and controversial concept.

5. As of 1984, life expectancy at birth of a black American female was 73.7 years as compared to 78.7 years for a white American female (figures for males are 65.6 and 71.8 years, respectively).   Part of this 5-year difference is due to differences in infant mortality, but the gap narrows progressively, so that, by age 85, a black woman has a slight edge, having an average 7.3 years of life expectancy, as compared to her white counterpart who has 6.5 years left. Black American men at 85 can expect to live an average 5.8 years, while white men have an average 5.1 year life expectancy.   There are no figures for average life expectancy at age 100.

When interpreting figures of life expectancy, it is important to know whether those figures are for birth, midlife, or late life. Although average life expectancy for American males and females at birth leapt 26 years, from 47 years in 1900 to 73 in 1980, there was an unimpressive 3-year increase in life expectancy at age 75 during that same time. Thus, Americans making it to age 75 in the year 1900 lived on the average to age 82, while the average person who was 75 in 1980 would live until age 85. There does not appear to have been any increase in maximal attainable life span, which is somewhere around 110 years.

Pearls:

1. You are only as old as you feel.

2. Some people are old at 18.

3. The cup of life is sweetest at the brim, the flavor is impaired as we reach the middle, and the dregs are made bitter so that we do not struggle when it is taken from our lips (Arabian proverb).

Pitfalls:

1. Not all cancers are more indolent in late life. Late-life thyroid carcinoma is usually of the aggressive anaplastic type. Nodular melanoma is aggressive at any age. Although some elderly patients may indeed have indolent solid tumors, others have tumors with similar growth rates to those in middle-aged people. Although breast cancer after menopause is less aggressive than in young women, it cannot be assumed that every old women with breast cancer will have a prolonged survival, and some studies describe shorter survival for women over 75. One of these oft-quoted studies was done in Sweden, where

there is a homogenous population that cannot be directly applied to the genetically heterogeneous American population. In addition, breast cancer survival studies generally do not hone in on the histologic subtypes. At least one expert believes that the relatively unusual small cell carcinoma is less aggressive than other histologic types, as demonstrated by the occurrence of remote metastases developing years later.

2. Although many people claim to be centenarians, there is not always written verification of their claims. Pockets of very old people have been described in various portions of the globe, including Ecuador, Soviet Georgia, and West Pakistan, where long-lived individuals have made all sorts of claims as to the reasons for their longevity. However, when documentation was sought, it was not forthcoming or did not exist. It has been concluded that many claims of extreme old age are due to various incentives--old-age pension, veneration, and regional publicity. There are few well-documented cases of people living to 110 years.

3. The main problem with being old is that you are young (O. Wilde).

References:

Adami H, Malker B, Holmberg L, Persson I, Stone B. The relation between survival and age at diagnosis in breast cancer. N Engl J Med 1986;315:559-563.

Cox EG. Breast cancer in the elderly. Clin Geriatr Med 1987;3:695-713.

Ershler WB. Why tumors grow more slowly in old people. JNCI 1986;77:837-839.

Fries JF. Aging, natural death, and the compression of morbidity. N Engl J Med 1980;303:130-135.

Haagensen CD. Diseases of the breast. Philadelphia: W.B. Saunders Co, 1986.

Leaf A. Long-lived populations: extreme old age. J Am Geriatr Soc 1982;30:485-487.

Suen KC, Lau LL, Yermakov V. Cancer and old age. An autopsy study of 3535 patients over 65 years old. Cancer 1974;33:1164-1168.

188   CASE STUDIES IN GERIATRICS

U.S. Department of Health and Human Services. National Center for Health
Statistics.   Health statistics on older persons, United States, 1986. DHHS
Publication No. (PHS) 87-1409:8.

Yin P, Shine M. Misinterpretations of increases in life expectancy in gerontology
textbooks. Gerontologist 1985;25:78-82.

PART II

**INTERPRETING LABORATORY VALUES
IN THE ELDERLY**

Problem 1.

A 70-year-old man has mild diabetes managed on diet. He reports persistently negative urine glucose using the Tes-Tape method at home. Fasting blood sugar is normal. Hemoglobin A_{1c} is 8% (N: less than 5%) and random blood glucose is 170 mg/dL (N: 70-118).

Questions:

1. What does the elevated glycosylated hemoglobin indicate in this clinical setting?

2. Give four possible explanations for the patient's persistently negative urine glucose.

Answers:

1. Although HbA_{1c} increases slightly with age, this patient's glycosylated hemoglobin level is clearly in the diabetic range, and reflects suboptimal control, probably after meals. Lack of glycemic control is confirmed by his frankly elevated random glucose level.

2. Glucose only "spills" into the urine when the tubular maximum (Tm) is reached, and this may vary from patient to patient. The renal threshold for glucose increases with age and it is not uncommon for high blood sugars, even in the high 200 range, to be unaccompanied by glycosuria. Blood glucose is occasionally over 250 mg/dL in elderly diabetics without glycosuria, so that the absence of glycosuria in the current patient would not be unexpected.

It is also possible that the patient is not performing the test correctly--he may be reading the test strip immediately instead of after the required 60 seconds have gone by, or he may be unable to read and interpret the chart correctly because of visual problems. Dilute urine can also reduce the sensitivity of urine monitoring techniques.

Drugs and other substances that produce false negative urine glucose results include salicylates, vitamin C, and levodopa. Aspirin and most other salicylates are metabolized to gentisic acid, a reducing agent that inhibits oxidation of the chromogen used in the glucose oxidase test (Tes-Tape, Diastix, Clinistix). Aspirin would have to be taken in relatively high doses (at least 2.5 grams per day) for this effect to occur. Levodopa, though a reducing metabolite, and vitamin C, can produce a false negative as well. Reducing agents tend to produce false-positive results when the copper reduction test (Clinitest) is used since, in this reaction, they reduce cupric sulfate (blue or green) to cuprous oxide (yellow or red), but some agents, such as cephalosporins and penicillins, can convert cupric sulfate to various copper sulfides, which can have a variety of colors that can be misinterpreted and sometimes considered falsely negative.

Home blood glucose monitoring should be done by the patient or family member whenever practical, regardless of the patient's age.

References:

Arnetz BB, Kallner A, Theorell T. The influence of aging on hemoglobin A_{1c}. J Gerontol 1982;37:648-650.

Butterfield WJH, Keen H, Whichelow MJ. Renal glucose threshold variations with age. Brit Med J 1967;4:505-507.

Rotblatt MD, Koda-Kimble MA. Review of drug interference with urine glucose tests. Diabetes Care 1987;10:103-110.

Rowe JW. Renal system. In: Rowe JW, Besdine RW. Geriatric Medicine. Boston: Little, Brown, 1988: 233-234.

Problem 2.

An 87-year-old woman is found to have a hematocrit of 34% and hemoglobin of 11 g/dL. Serum iron and total iron binding capacity (TIBC) are low. Serum ferritin is 40 ng/mL (N: greater than 30). She takes enteric-coated aspirin for chronic low back pain due to lumbosacral degenerative disc disease.

Questions:

1. Is the patient anemic?

2. How can the normal ferritin and low serum iron be reconciled?

3. What is the meaning of the low serum iron in combination with low iron binding capacity?

Answers:

1. Normal values for hemoglobin and hematocrit do not change with age. The patient in question is anemic.

2. Normal laboratory ranges for ferritin reflect iron status in healthy, nonelderly adults. Serum ferritin rises with age, since iron stores increase with age, particularly in women. In addition, ferritin can be elevated in chronic inflammatory conditions, which stimulate and activate the reticulo-endothelial system. Since such chronic conditions often exist in late life, ferritin may be misleadingly high. Thus, a "low normal" serum ferritin in an elderly individual may actually indicate critically low iron stores, a situation that has been documented in studies that have included bone marrow evaluation. On the other hand, serum iron is always low when marrow stores are absent.

3. In general, low iron and low TIBC indicate anemia of chronic disease, and not iron deficiency. However, TIBC depends on adequate serum proteins. Iron is required for protein synthesis, which may be impaired in elderly patients, particularly in the setting of acute or chronic illness.

References:

Casale G, Bonora C, Migliavacca A, et al. Serum ferritin and aging. Age Ageing 1981;10:119-122.

Htoo MSH, Kofkoff RL, Freedman ML. Erythrocyte parameters in the elderly: an argument against new geriatric normal values. J Amer Geriatr Soc 1979;27:547-551.

Reed AH, Cannon DC, Winkelman JW, et al. Estimation of normal ranges from a controlled sample survey. Clin Chem 1972;18:57-66.

Sharma JC, Ray SN. Value of serum ferritin as an index of iron deficiency in elderly anemic patients. Age Ageing 1984;13:248-250.

Problem 3.

A 72-year-old woman is found to have a regular heart rate of 108. There is no goiter, palpable thyroid nodule, or exophthalmos. She drinks 8 cups of coffee per day. T_4 = 10.8 μg/dL (N = 6.2-13.2) and T_3RU = 31% (N = 20-32). T_3RIA = 259 ng/dL (N = 110-250). EKG reveals sinus rhythm.

Questions:

1. On the basis of the laboratory values given, how certain is the diagnosis of hyperthyroidism?

2. What is the most reliable test that can be done to confirm the diagnosis of hyperthyroidism?

3. How can the elevated hormone levels be reconciled with the paucity of physical findings?

Answers:

1. In view of the sole elevation of T_3RIA, the patient could have T_3 toxicosis. Although T_3 is only mildly elevated, T_3 levels are frequently lower in apparently healthy elderly, and it has been suggested by some that the upper limits of normal be age-adjusted to reflect this. In accord with age-adjusted norms, this patient's T_3 would be unequivocally elevated. Her mild symptoms nonetheless require further testing. To begin with, her blood tests should be repeated.

2. The TRH stimulation test is the most sensitive test that can be used to confirm the diagnosis of hyperthyroidism. The response of TSH to TRH infusion can be blunted in healthy elderly individuals and so it must be interpreted with caution. However, in primary hyperthyroidism, TSH curve is flat, so that even in the elderly the test is reliable in this clinical situation.

3. Grave's disease with its classic stigmata (goiter, exophthalmos, and dermopathy) is an uncommon cause of hyperthyroidism in people over 70 years of age. Hyperthyroidism in the elderly is more commonly associated with multinodular gland, a functioning nodule, or thyroiditis. Diffuse, palpable goiter is uncommon.

References:

Gambert SR, Tsitouras PD. Effect of age on thyroid hormone physiology and function. J Amer Geriatr Soc 1985;33:360-365.

Gregerman RI. Intrinsic physiologic variables. In: Ingbar SH, Braverman LE. Werner's The Thyroid. Philadelphia: Lippincot, 1986:361-381.

Schimmel M, Utiger RD. Thyroidal and peripheral production of thyroid hormones: review of recent findings and their clinical implications. Ann Intern Med 1977;87:760-768.

Problem 4.

A 78-year-old man, who has been well all his life, is found to have a total serum protein of 8.6 g/dL (N = 6.3-8.2) and albumin of 3.9 g/dL (N = 3.7-5.1) on routine chemistry screen. His physical examination, CBC, urinalysis, and other blood chemistries are normal.

Questions:

1. What is a possible explanation for his elevated serum protein?

2. What treatment plan should be recommended?

Answers:

1. At least 3% of people over the age of 70 are found to have "benign monoclonal gammopathy" (BMG)--a monoclonal protein in the serum in concentrations of less than 3 gm/dL, and without physical or laboratory evidence of multiple myeloma, macroglobulinemia, or related diseases. This phenomenon is far more common among the elderly than among younger adults. Polyclonal gammopathy would also cause elevated serum proteins and could be caused by a chronic inflammatory process or smoldering infection, but the patient with a polyclonal gammopathy would be more likely to feel ill than a patient with BMG.

2. Immunoelectrophoresis and urine for Bence-Jones protein should be done. If BMG is confirmed, no treatment is required. However, careful followup is essential since nearly 20% of affected individuals who survive for 10 years develop malignant lymphoproliferative diseases. Elderly patients with BMG are less likely than younger adults to go on to develop such diseases since 40% will die of unrelated causes before the disease has had time to make its appearance. Because of the malignant potential of "benign" monoclonal gammopathy, some investigators prefer the term, "monoclonal gammopathy of undetermined significance."

References:

Hallen J. Frequency of "abnormal" serum globulins (M-components) in the aged. Acta Med Scand 1963;173:737-744.

Kyle RA. "Benign" monoclonal gammopathy: a misnomer? JAMA 1984;251:1849-1854.

Problem 5.

A 78-year-old woman with congestive heart failure and chronic atrial fibrillation has been taking digoxin 0.25 mg per day for several years and furosemide for 6 months. She now has junctional bradycardia (rate = 44). Digoxin level is 0.8 ng/mL (N: 0.8-2.0) and serum potassium is normal. Serum creatinine is normal and unchanged from last year, when her digoxin level was 0.9.

Questions:

1. What are the possible explanations for her bradycardia?

2. Why do such low serum digoxin levels exist in the face of her "nongeriatric" dose?

Answers:

1. It is very possible that the patient's cardiac disease has deteriorated to the extent that her diseased myocardium has become overly sensitive to the effects of digoxin. The arrhythmia may not represent digoxin toxicity at all, but is an arrhythmia of the diseased heart itself. Another possibility is that she has developed magnesium depletion. Diuretics that waste potassium are also capable of depleting the system of magnesium. Digoxin acts by inhibiting sodium-potassium adenosine triphosphatase (NaK-ATPase), increasing intracellular sodium and making more calcium available for activation of myocardial and conducting tissue. Not only is magnesium needed for activation of NaK-ATPase, but magnesium depletion potentiates intracellular potassium loss and increases myocardial cell uptake of digoxin, thereby increasing the risk of digoxin toxicity. In this setting, as in other situations where the myocardium is ultrasensitive to digoxin (such as hypokalemia), toxicity can be manifest in the face of normal to subtherapeutic digoxin levels. Serum magnesium levels are not terribly accurate and red cell magnesium levels should be obtained if possible. If magnesium status cannot be determined but if depletion is suspected in the face of a refractory dig-toxic rhythm, magnesium should be given empirically. Hypercalcemia, another problem that can lead to dig-toxic arrhythmias, can occur in susceptible individuals given oral furosemide without salt loading.

Although NaK-ATPase activity may be reduced with age, the aged myocardium, in the absence of disease, has not been clinically demonstrated to be more sensitive to the effects of digoxin.

2. A lower than expected digoxin level can indicate lack of patient compliance, malabsorption or excessive degradation of digoxin, or change to a less bioavailable brand or preparation of digoxin.

The average therapeutic dose of digoxin declines with age because of declining renal function. However, there is great interindividual variation in serum digoxin levels. This heterogeneity is enhanced in the geriatric population because "age-related" decline in renal function is very variable. The dose of digoxin has to be strictly individualized in all patients. Just as there is a risk of overdosing the elderly, adequate dose should not be avoided because of unconfirmed fears of renal decline.

References:

Aronson JK. Indications for the measurement of plasma digoxin concentrations. Drugs 1983;26:230-242.

Smith TW. Pharmacokinetics, bioavailability and serum levels of cardiac glycosides. J Amer Coll Cardiol 1985;5:43A-50A.

Surawicz B. Factors affecting tolerance to digitalis. J Amer Coll Cardiol 1985;5:69A-81A.

Problem 6.

A 78-year-old woman complains of fatigue, stiffness in the shoulders and neck, recent onset of bitemporal head pains, "bumps" and redness in the temples, and an episode of transient visual loss in one eye. Erythrocyte sedimentation rate (ESR) = 24 mm/hr.

Questions:

1. What is the diagnosis?

2. Does an age adjustment need to be made for ESR?

3. Given the probable diagnosis, how could the sedimentation rate be explained?

Answers:

1. The diagnosis, made on clinical grounds, is temporal arteritis.

2. ESR rises slightly with age. Current consensus is that, over the age of 50 years, the upper limits of normal should be 20 mm/hr for men and 30 mm/hr for women. However, ESR is usually under 20 mm/hr in healthy elderly individuals. Autopsy studies have demonstrated that the frank elevations seen in some asymptomatic individuals may actually indicate occult disease that does not present itself during life. In short, elevated ESR probably has the same significance in old age that it does in younger adulthood, and the clinical situation should be the final determination of how aggressive the workup should be.

3. Normal ESR has been reported to occur in patients with biopsy-proven temporal arteritis, a phenomenon that has not been fully explained. While this has been reported to occur in fewer than 9% of cases, the actual proportion could well be much higher, because the finding of a normal ESR is likely to discourage a physician from pursuing the diagnosis further. Congestive heart failure, if present, may lower ESR. In addition, the use of nonsteroidal anti-inflammatory agents could theoretically lower ESR in this setting by reducing the inflammatory response. Patients diagnosed with temporal arteritis are likely to have been taking analgesics for headaches, joint pains, and other discomforts. Other factors that can falsely lower the ESR include delay in processing the specimen and overdilution of the specimen with anticoagulant. Finally, depending on the laboratory method used, the test may lack sufficient sensitivity if fibrinogen levels are only mildly elevated.

References:

Gibson II. The value of erythrocyte sedimentation rate in the aged. Gerontol Clin 1972;14:185-190.

Hunder GG, Hazleman BL. Giant cell arteritis and polymyalgia rheumatica. In: Kelley WN, Harris ED, Ruddy S, et al. Textbook of Rheumatology. Philadelphia: WB Saunders, 1985:1166-1173.

Sox HC, Liang MH. The erythrocyte sedimentation rate. Ann Intern Med 1986;104:515-523.

Sparrow D, Rowe JW, Silbert JE. Cross-sectional and longitudinal changes in the erythrocyte sedimentation rate in men. J Gerontol 1981;36:180-184.

Wong RL, Korn JH.   Temporal arteritis without an elevated erythrocyte sedimentation rate. Am J Med 1986;80:959-964.

Problem 7.

An 83-year-old woman undergoes a workup for progressive memory loss over 2 years. Neurologic examination is normal except for decreased vibratory sensation using a 256 cycles-per-second tuning fork. Hematocrit = 39%, hemoglobin = 13.7 g%, mean corpuscular volume = 92 μm^3 (N = 90±9), serum B_{12} = 120 pg/mL (N = 200-900). Stool guaiac is positive.

Questions:

1. Of what use is the Schilling test in this patient?

2. What are the possible diagnoses?

3. What are the most sensitive indicators of B_{12} deficiency anemia?

Answers:

1. Symptomatic vitamin B_{12} deficiency may exist in the absence of anemia, but the diagnosis is often difficult to ascertain, since many patients with low serum B_{12} levels have a normal Schilling test. The accuracy of the standard Schilling test has been questioned by investigators who have found that food cobalamin is absorbed poorly by some patients with a normal Schilling test, which measures the absorption of free cobalamin. This subtle malabsorption seems to occur in the absence of full-blown autoimmune atrophic gastritis. Serum measurements of B_{12} are currently a subject of controversy. Low levels have been attributed to reduced levels of transcobalamin II, a serum binding protein for B_{12}, found to be low in 10% of elderly patients who are hematologically normal. On the other hand, low B_{12} levels may represent preclinical pernicious anemia due to a subtle malabsorption syndrome.

It is extremely difficult to collect an adequate 24-hour urine specimen in an elderly woman with dementia, making a Schilling test impractical and possibly misleading. In view of this and the other difficulties, the most sensible solution in such cases is to omit the Schilling test and give empiric treatment with parenteral B_{12}.

2. Progressive memory loss without other psychiatric abnormalities in an elderly person is more typical of Alzheimer's disease than dementia due to B_{12} deficiency. The latter is often complicated by other psychiatric or physical symptoms. The co-occurrence of mildly impaired vibratory sensation without impaired proprioception may be a normal aging phenomenon. The laboratory findings are not particularly helpful, since low B_{12} levels are common in patients with Alzheimer's disease, without a pathogenetic association, and in apparently normal elderly. However, the low level could indicate early B_{12} deficiency, and, in view of her memory loss, a trial of vitamin B_{12} is indicated.

3. In true B_{12} deficiency, the first abnormality in the hematologic picture is the appearance of hypersegmented polymorphonuclear leukocytes on peripheral smear. Elevated mean corpuscular volume occurs in pernicious anemia before frank anemia sets in, but MCV has been reported to increase slightly with normal aging, and is elevated in a variety of other conditions. Also, mixed microcytic and macrocytic anemias are common in the elderly so that the MCV could actually be normal in this setting. Although this particular patient was not anemic, she was found to have iron deficiency and an unusual gastric lesion--a leiomyoma. Many gastric abnormalities can impair B_{12} absorption, but structural lesions probably are far less common than atrophic gastritis.

References:

Carmel R, Sinow RM, Siegel ME, Samloff IM. Food cobalamin malabsorption occurs frequently in patients with unexplained low serum cobalamin levels. Arch Intern Med 1988;148:1715-1719.

Helman N, Rubenstein LS. The effects of age, sex, and smoking on erythrocytes and leukocytes. Am J Clin Path 1975;63:35-44.

Lindenbaum J, Healton EB, Savage DG, Brust JCM, Garrett TJ, Podell ER, et al. Neuropsychiatric disorders caused by cobalamin deficiency in the absence of anemia or macrocytosis. N Engl J Med 1988;318:1720-1728.

Marcus DL, Grinblat J, Freedman ML. Transcobalamin II levels in a geriatric population with low vitamin B_{12}. The Gerontologist 24:98, 1984 (abstract).

Problem 8.

An 86-year-old woman has a random blood sugar (plasma glucose) of 160 mg/dL. She says she is feeling well.

Questions:

1. What is the significance of the laboratory finding in an elderly patient?

2. What should be done?

Answers:

1. Although impaired glucose tolerance occurs in as many as 50% of people 65 and older, glucose intolerance is not considered a normal aging phenomenon and the official National Diabetes Data Group (NDDG) criteria for the diagnosis of diabetes mellitus in the elderly are the same as in younger adults. A random glucose of 160 is strongly suggestive of diabetes at any age, but the actual diagnosis rests on confirmatory testing.

It is important to realize that current criteria are very conservative and perhaps insufficiently sensitive for the very old, who would be classified as diabetic by World Health Organization criteria (2-hour value on oral glucose tolerance test [GTT] of greater than 140). The NDDG wished to reduce the rate of false-positive diagnoses, which may result in employment and insurance bias, and overtreatment.

2. Drugs interfering with glucose metabolism, such as thiazides or glucocorticoids, should be discontinued if possible. Plasma glucose should be determined after a 10- to 16-hour fast. If the value is 140 mg/dL or more on two determinations, or if a random glucose is 200 mg/dL or more, the criteria for diabetes are met and further testing, such as a glucose tolerance test, is not required.

If fasting glucose if technically normal but the patient has symptoms and signs suggestive of diabetes, such as monilial vaginitis, intertrigo, peripheral neuropathy, or microangiopathy on funduscopic examination, glucose tolerance testing should be considered, keeping in mind that oral glucose load produces greater elevations in blood glucose than does a meal.

Treatment of mild hyperglycemia in the elderly should consist of diet, exercise, and weight loss if indicated. Drug treatment should be reserved for those with overt diabetes, and, depending on the reliability and symptoms of the patient, should be conservative. The immediate symptoms of hypoglycemia may be subtle or absent in those elderly whose counterregulatory mechanisms are blunted, and the effects of hypoglycemia in the elderly may be more serious than in the young.

References:

Goldberg AP, Andres R, Bierman EL. Diabetes mellitus in the elderly. In: Andres R, Bierman EL, Hazzard WR. Principles of Geriatric Medicine. New York: McGraw-Hill, 1985:750-763.

Harris MI, Hadden WC, Knowler WC et al. International criteria for the diagnosis of diabetes and impaired glucose tolerance. Diabetes Care 1985;8:562-567.

National Diabetes Data Group: Classification and diagnosis of diabetes mellitus and other categories of glucose intolerance. Diabetes 1979;28:1039-1057.

Nelson RL. Oral glucose tolerance test: indications and limitations. Mayo Clin Proc 1988;63:263-269.

Problem 9.

A 94-year-old man suffers from severe peripheral vascular disease and is being treated for leg pain and a small ischemic ulcer on his big toe. His appetite is poor and he is losing weight. His serum albumin is 2.9 g/dL.

Questions:

1. Is his serum albumin normal for his age?

2. What is the significance of a low albumin in an elderly person?

Answers:

1. Serum protein levels do decline slightly with age, but, in healthy elderly, they should fall within the normal range. This patient's albumin level is definitely low. Protein synthesis proceeds normally in the healthy elderly if protein intake is sufficient, but levels of serum albumin are exquisitely sensitive to protein intake and to an unexpectedly wide range of illnesses. For example, one investigator demonstrated that low serum albumin correlated with coronary artery disease. Although no physiologic age change in protein metabolism has been demonstrated in the living human organism, subtle cellular changes may occur.

2. The sensitivity of serum albumin to a range of illnesses in the elderly has prompted some observers to refer to this measurement as a "negative acute phase reactant." Although it may be a sensitive sign of illness, serum albumin probably is even less specific than the sensitive but nonspecific erythrocyte sedimentation rate. Low serum albumin reduces colloid osmotic pressure and allows "third-spacing" to occur in severe renal or hepatic disease, but in patients like the present one it is a sign rather than a cause of clinical problems.

Chronically low serum albumin in patients taking drugs that are protein-bound should result in higher free, active fraction of the agent. Increased sensitivity to the drug might occur, but free drug is also more rapidly excreted and the steady state concentration and sensitivity to the drug may not be significantly altered for this reason.

References:

Campion EW, deLabry LO, Glynn RJ. The effect of age on serum albumin in healthy males: report from the normative aging study. J Gerontol 1988;43:M18-M20.

Gersovitz M, Hunro HN, Young VR. Albumin synthesis in young and elderly subjects using a new stable isotope methodology: response to level of protein intake. Metabolism 1980;29:1075-1086.

Greenblatt DJ. Reduced serum albumin concentration in the elderly: a report from the Boston Collaborative Drug Surveillance Program. J Amer Geriatr Soc 1979;27:20-22.

Greenblatt DJ, Sellers EM, Shader RI. Drug disposition in old age. N Engl J Med 1982:306:1081-1087.

Hodkinson HM. Biochemical diagnosis of the elderly. New York: John Wiley, 1977.

Pickhart L. Increased ratio of free fatty acids to albumin during normal aging and in patients with coronary heart disease. Atherosclerosis 1983;46:21-28.

213

Problem 10.

A 69-year-old man complains of inability to obtain and maintain an erection with his sexual partner. His erectile difficulties seem to have come on after his wife died 4 years ago. Neurologic and genital examinations are normal. At his insistence, a testosterone determination is done. Total testosterone = 264 ng/dL (N = 360-900) and free testosterone = 4.0 ng/dL (N = 5.1-41.0). Except for a hematocrit of 39%, other blood tests are normal.

Questions:

1. What is the meaning of the low testosterone level?

2. What are the possible explanations for his erectile difficulties?

Answers:

1. Average testosterone levels of an elderly male population are lower than levels in younger groups, but longitudinal studies of healthy men have demonstrated no real decline. Since the level of total testosterone is dependent on the level of sex hormone binding globulin, which may increase with age and disease, free testosterone level is more reflective of testosterone status. Also, since testosterone is secreted in a pulsatile fashion, a single sample may not be reflective of overall status. No age-adjusted range has been determined and there is wide interindividual variation in levels.

With age, the number of sexual events declines, the time to attain erection increases, the refractory period required to next erection increases, and the erection may be less firm. There is, however, no strong correlation between sexual activity and serum testosterone levels, with both serum testosterone levels and sexual activity correlating better with general health than with age alone. Moreover, a threshold of serum testosterone has not been determined, below which sexual dysfunction occurs.

2. The incidence of impotence increases dramatically with age over 45, with over 50% of men suffering from impotence after the age of 75. This may be due to a variety of disorders, drugs, and psychologic factors. This patient was not taking drugs known to affect sexual function, such as anticholinergic agents, antidepressants, alcohol, or central nervous system depressants, and did not have physical evidence of vascular, endocrinologic, or neurologic disease. However, the low hematocrit should prompt a careful workup, since underlying disease correlates with low testosterone levels and sexual dysfunction.

Although psychogenic factors are less likely than other factors to be to blame in elderly men, in whom organic explanations are often found, psychologic factors could have been operating in this patient in whom the onset of his problem more or less coincided with the death of his wife.

References:

Davidson JM, Chen JJ, Crapo L, Gray GD, Greenleaf WJ, Catania JA. Hormonal changes and sexual function in aging men. J Clin Endocrinol Metab 1983;57:71-77.

Harman SM, Tsitouras PD.   Reproductive hormones in aging men. I. Measurement of sex steroids, basal luteinizing hormone, and Leydig cell response to human chorionic gonadotropin.   J Clin Endocrinol Metab 1980;51:35-40.

Pfeiffer E, Verwoerdt A, Wang H.   Sexual behavior in aged men and women. Arch Gen Psychiatr 1968;19:753-758.

Tsitouras PD, Martin CE, Harman SM. Relationship of serum testosterone to sexual activity in healthy elderly men. J Gerontol 1982;37:288-293.

Problem 11.

The following patients have been evaluated and found to have a thyroid stimulating hormone (TSH) level of 12 μU/mL (N = 0.8-4.8).

a 78-year-old healthy woman
a 78-year-old woman with fatigue
a 78-year-old woman with dementia
a 78-year-old woman with a 10-pound weight gain

What should be done?

Answer:

On routine screening, and excluding patients with known hypothyroidism, TSH may be greater than 10 uU/mL in more than 7% of women over 60 years of age, a prevalence that increases still further in populations over 75, and in institutionalized elderly. The prevalence is somewhat lower in men than in women. Elevated TSH may be accompanied by normal or low levels of thyroid hormones.

A patient with a high TSH in the face of persistently normal serum levels of thyroid hormone is said to have the "failing thyroid syndrome," a condition in which increased pituitary secretion of TSH maintains homeostasis in someone who may have subclinical thyroid dysfunction. If the patient is asymptomatic, treatment is probably not indicated. However, thyroid function tests should be performed periodically since thyroid function may decline further with time. Symptoms of hypothyroidism are so nonspecific in old age that they cannot be relied upon as warning signs.

If thyroxine levels are low (confirmed by calculation of free thyroxine index), it is generally recommended to treat the patient with the lowest possible dose of L-thyroxine (usual starting dose is 25 micrograms per day). However, treating hypothyroidism of this mild degree is unlikely to reverse symptoms such as dementia, fatigue, or weight gain, which are often due to other factors in elderly patients. Because thyroid replacement therapy may exacerbate angina, cardiac arrhythmias, and bone resorption, some clinicians elect to follow, rather than treat, asymptomatic patients with mild chemical hypothyroidism.

References:

Livingston EH, Hershman JM, Sawin CT, Yoshikawa TT. Prevalence of thyroid disease and abnormal thyroid tests in older hospitalized and ambulatory persons. J Amer Geriatr Soc 1987;35:109-114.

Sawin CT, Chopra D, Azizi F, et al. The aging thyroid: increased prevalence of elevated serum thyrotropin levels in the elderly. JAMA 1979;242:247-250.

Problem 12.

An 85-year-old man is hospitalized with fever, lethargy, and a urinary tract infection. Cultures are drawn and treatment will include an aminoglycoside antibiotic. The patient weighs 70 kg and his serum creatinine is 1.0 mg/dL (N = 0.1-1.1).

Questions:

1. How may the patient's creatinine be applied in calculating the dosage of a drug such as gentamicin?

2. What should be the initial dose of gentamicin in this patient?

Answers:

1. In the elderly, serum creatinine correlates poorly with creatinine clearance and cannot be relied upon to calculate dosages of renally excreted drugs that have a narrow therapeutic-to-toxic ratio. On the average, glomerular filtration, and hence creatinine clearance, declines by 50% between the ages of 20 and 70 years. At the same time, creatinine production declines with age, because of decreased muscle mass, offsetting the reduction in creatinine clearance, and serum creatinine does not increase unless renal function is severely impaired. There is wide interindividual variation in age-related decline in renal function, so that many old people have creatinine clearance in the youthful range. Thus, popular formulas used to estimate creatinine clearance by age and serum creatinine can be very misleading.

Age-related decline in renal function may have no clinical significance, since production of various renally excreted endogenous substances may decline concomitantly, and internal homeostasis is maintained. The problem arises when exogenous substances such as aminoglycoside antibiotics are administered. If it is impractical to collect a 24-hour urine to measure creatinine clearance, impaired renal function should be assumed until proven otherwise, and dose adjustments of potentially toxic drugs should be made on the basis of serum drug levels.

2. The initial dose of gentamicin in this patient should be 1 mg per kg body weight, or 70 mg, as it would be for a young adult with normal renal function. Aminoglycosides are not tightly bound to serum proteins and distribute widely, so that equilibrium with the extracellular compartment is not reached until a day or so after treatment is initiated. During the period of equilibration, the patient's renal function has less of an impact on the plasma levels achieved than during maintenance therapy, when it has a critical impact.

Although toxicity must be avoided, it is also important not to err on the side of underdosing when treating serious illness, a problem that sometimes (though not often) occurs when physicians are overly cautious in prescribing for elderly patients.

References:

Lindeman RD, Tobin JD, Shock NW. Longitudinal studies on the rate of decline in renal function with age. J Amer Geriatr Soc 1985;33:278-285.

Lye MDW. The milieu interieur and aging. In: Brocklehurst JC, ed. Textbook of geriatric medicine and gerontology. Edinburgh: Churchill Livingstone, 1985:201-229.

Rowe JW, Andres R, Tobin JD, Norris AH, Shock NW. The effect of age on creatinine clearance in men: a cross-sectional and longitudinal study. J Gerontol 1976;31:155-163.

Problem 13.

A 78-year-old woman has developed progessive memory loss and confusion over a period of 4 years, and is thought to have Alzheimer's disease (AD). There are no other abnormalities on neurologic examination, and blood tests are normal. Computerized tomography (CT scan) of the brain with and without contrast shows cortical atrophy with ventricles enlarged out of proportion to sulcal widening, but is otherwise normal. The patient is taking no medications.

Questions:

1. What information has this radiologic test contributed to the diagnosis?

2. What other testing might be considered?

Answer:

1. The CT scan has ruled out a reversible structural lesion but has otherwise not contributed to the diagnosis of AD. Cortical atrophy may be present in cognitively normal elderly people and is considered a normal finding. The diagnosis of Alzheimer's disease is best made with a careful history and physical examination.

2. Ventricles may be disproportionately enlarged in normal aging and in AD, but if sulci are minimally enlarged, or if ventricles are greatly enlarged, hydrocephalus may be present and magnetic resonance imaging (MRI) should be considered. Normal pressure hydrocephalus (NPH) is a rare cause of senile dementia, in which subarachnoid outflow of cerebrospinal fluid is impaired. This disease generally presents with a gait disorder and behavioral changes such as apathy, social disinhibition, and other symptoms that are less characteristic of AD, making the diagnosis unlikely in this case. However, NPH is potentially reversible, and if it is suspected, MRI should be done because it may demonstrate periventricular edema and can help to identify patients who will benefit from a shunt procedure. Lumbar puncture with removal of a small amount of CSF may relieve symptoms temporarily and strongly suggests the diagnosis. Neither test was indicated in this case because the disproportionate enlargement of the ventricles was slight.

The diagnosis of NPH should not be made lightly. Postoperative morbidity of a shunt procedure is substantial, and elderly patients tend to respond less well to the procedure than do younger patients.

References:

Ford CV, Winter J. Computerized axial tomograms and dementia in elderly patients, J Gerontol 1981;36:164-169.

Gerard G, Weisberg LA. Magnetic resonance imaging in adult white matter disorders and hydrocephalus. Sem Neurol 1986;6:17-23.

Horowitz GR. What is a complete work-up for dementia? Clin Geriatr Med 1988;4:163-180.

McKhann G, Drachman D, Folstein M, Katzman R, Price D, Stadlan EM. Clinical diagnosis of Alzheimer's disease: report of the NINCDS-ADRDA work group under the auspices of the Department of Health and Human Services Task Force on Alzheimer's Disease. Neurology 1984;34:939-944.

Problem 14.

A 79-year-old woman with severe emphysema is found to have sinus tachycardia and paroxysmal supraventricular tachycardia. Serum T_4 and T_3RU studies are normal, but T_3RIA is elevated in two of three determinations, and TSH level is very low. Thyrotropin-releasing-hormone (TRH) stimulation test is done and reveals

Time	Baseline	30 min	45 min	60 min
TSH (μU/mL)	0.3	0.4	0.4	0.3

(Normal unstimulated TSH = 0.8-4.8)

Questions:

1. Is the TRH test helpful in this situation?

2. Is the TRH test helpful in diagnosing hypothyroidism?

Answers:

1.   Although the TRH test is usually not necessary in the diagnosis of hyperthyroidism, a confirmatory test is important in this case since her cardiac arrhythmia has two potential causes and the clinical elements must be carefully delineated.   Caution has been advised in interpreting the results of the TRH test in the elderly because some studies have demonstrated a blunted response of TSH to the administration of TRH in aged subjects.   However, other studies have failed to demonstrate a blunted response, and the reasons for the discrepancy may include gender differences, as well as lack of uniformity among subjects and inclusion criteria in the studies.   Despite the possibility that the response is blunted in some elderly, this patient's TSH response curve is completely "flat," and is consistent with hyperthyroidism.

2.   The elderly patient with primary hypothyroidism exhibits the same exaggerated response of TSH to TRH stimulation as that seen in younger hypothyroid patients.   However, the TRH test is rarely indicated in the diagnosis of hypothyroidism, since almost all cases in the elderly are due to primary thyroid failure and are accompanied by an elevated TSH.   The TRH test should only be done if there is a suspicion of pituitary hypothyroidism, an extremely rare clinical condition.

References:

Gambert SR, Tsitouras PD. Effect of age on thyroid hormone physiology and function. J Amer Geriatr Soc 1985;33:360-365.

Kolesnick RN, Gershengorn MC.   Thyrotropin-releasing hormone and the pituitary. Am J Med 1985;79:729-739.

Snyder PJ, Utiger RD. Responses to thyrotropin releasing hormone in normal man. J Clin Endocrinol Metab 1972;34:380-385.

Problem 15.

A 66-year-old obese woman has been taking liothyronine (Cytomel) for many years. Her serum T_4 = 7.8 μg/dL, and T_3RU = 24%, both normal values. She has stable exertional angina. At age 30 she received "iodine" for a goiter.

Questions:

1. Is her thyroid medication indicated?

2. Why is she taking it?

Answers:

1. This patient does not need thyroid medication. If she were truly hypothyroid, her serum T_4 level would be extremely low, since replacement with liothyronine (synthetic T_3) would suppress her pituitary-thyroid axis. Her thyroid gland is functioning normally because, despite pituitary suppression, normal amounts of thyroid hormone are being produced. Moreover, her serum T_3RIA was found to be elevated at 231 ng/dL (N = 90-225). T_3 levels are often decreased in late life because of decreased peripheral conversion of T_4 to T_3, a phenomenon that occurs in many clinical situations. For this reason, a mildly elevated T_3RIA increases in significance in an elderly person.

It was once considered more physiologic to treat with T_3 than with thyroxine (T_4), since the former is the active form of the hormone. However, thyroxine is adequately converted to T_3 in the body and is the drug of choice. Preparations containing T_3 should actually be avoided in the elderly since T_3 is rapidly absorbed and rapidly disappears from plasma. The daily rush of hormone that occurs is thought to have an excessive cardiostimulatory effect that is to be avoided older patients.

Withdrawal of Cytomel resulted in maintenance of the euthyroid state in this patient, but angina persisted. She did not gain more weight.

2. Many elderly patients who are taking thyroid hormone for "hypothyroidism" are actually euthyroid. In some, the diagnosis was made in the remote past, using laboratory methods now known to be nonspecific, such as basal metabolism rate, protein-bound iodine, or clinical clues that are notoriously unreliable in the elderly.   Unless the method of diagnosis can be ascertained, it may be fruitful to lower the dose of thyroid hormone and follow the TSH level. If the patient is found to be euthyroid, the next task is to convince the patient of this, which is not always easy!

References:

Feit H. Thyroid function in the elderly. Clin Geriatr Med 1988;4:151-161.

Schimmel M, Utiger RD. Thyroidal and peripheral production of thyroid hormones: review of recent findings and their clinical implications. Ann Intern Med 1977;87:760-768.

Problem 16.

A 76-year-old woman with no history of liver disease or blood transfusion complains of fatigue. Laboratory evaluation has revealed persistent elevation of transaminase enzymes (SGOT = 60 IU [N: less than 40] and SGPT = 90 IU [N: less than 40]). There are no stigmata of liver disease, and alkaline phosphatase, bilirubin, and ferritin are normal. Hepatitis B surface antibody (HepB$_s$Ab) is positive. Hepatitis A IgG and IgM antibodies are negative. Antinuclear antibody (ANA) is negative and antimitochondrial antibody (AMA) is positive at a titer of 1:640. She reports that her brother, who was a nonalcoholic, died of "cirrhosis" when he was in his forties.

Questions:

1. Why are the liver function tests abnormal?

2. What alternative explanation exists for the positive AMA?

Answers:

1. Nonspecific liver abnormalities are a common histologic finding at autopsy in elderly patients with no known history of liver disease, but are not associated with elevation of liver enzymes. Alkaline phosphatase is occasionally elevated in women and thought to be due to nonspecific bone disease. The positive HepB$_s$Ab indicates prior infection with hepatitis B virus; evidence of past infection with this virus is present in 30% of elderly people with no history of clinical infection or transfusion. The presence of antibody indicates that a previous hepatitis B infection has been arrested so that chronic disease could not be due to this virus. Although enteral infection with non-A non-B virus is theoretically possible, it is exceedingly rare.

The patient may have early primary biliary cirrhosis (PBC), as indicated by the elevation of AMA. PBC that presents in late life usually is detected when automated chemistry screening reveals abnormal liver function tests, and the disease tends to run a benign course that is compatible with a normal life span. The family history of "cirrhosis" is of interest, since PBC probably has a genetic component, but PBC is rare in men. The normal ferritin level rules out hemochromatosis, another genetic disease affecting the liver.

2. Low titers of one or more autoantibodies (rheumatoid factor, ANA, AMA, antiparietal cell, antithyroid, biologic false positive VDRL, and others) are found in as many as 30 to 40% of elderly people over the age of 80, in the absence of overt autoimmune disease. The titer of AMA in this patient is considered "borderline," and not definitely indicative of PBC. Still, no other explanation for her liver function abnormalities exists.

The explanations for the age-related increase in autoantibodies include decreased suppressor T-cell activity, exposure of previously hidden cellular antigens, and the accumulation of substances in the body that nonspecifically stimulate B cells to produce antibodies. This increase in low titer autoantibodies is not associated with a general increase in overt autoimmune disease.

References:

Blandford G, Zeitz HJ, Samter M. Immunology in old age. In: Samter M, ed. Immunological diseases. 4th ed. Boston: Little, Brown, 1988:2036-2044.

Finkelstein MS, Freedman, ML, Shenkman L, Krugman S. Evidence of prior hepatitis B and hepatitis A virus infection in an ambulatory geriatric population. J Gerontol 1981;36:302-305.

Lehmann AB, Bassendine MF, James OFW. Is primary biliary cirrhosis a different disease in the elderly? Gerontology 1985;31:186-194.

Roll J, Bayer JL, Barry D, Klatskin G. The prognostic importance of clinical and histologic features in asymptomatic and symptomatic primary biliary cirrhosis. N Engl J Med 1983;308:1-7.

Problem 17.

A 90-year-old man with venous insufficiency has a large, chronic stasis ulcer on his lower leg. Plasma zinc level is 100 μg/dL (normal is greater than 110). He takes furosemide 40 mg per day. Is zinc therapy indicated?

Answer:

Determination of zinc status is difficult because plasma measurements are insensitive, highly variable, and correlate poorly with tissue levels. Some studies indicate a decline in blood levels of zinc with age, possibly because of inadequate intake or the presence of disease and drugs known to impair zinc status. True zinc deficiency may cause impaired taste and smell, impaired wound healing, and abnormal immune function, problems that also happen to increase in prevalence with age. However, despite the presence of suboptimal zinc status in certain elderly, zinc supplementation has not been shown to improve idiopathic hyposmia, and wound healing is not accelerated by zinc therapy unless frankly abnormal zinc status is present.

Immune function may be enhanced by pharmacologic doses of zinc, but such therapy should not be given for prolonged periods because zinc excess can result in copper deficiency and possibly other problems as well.

Furosemide accelerates renal loss of zinc and theoretically could impair this patient's zinc status. A short course (less than 2 months) of oral zinc therapy would not cause harm and might speed healing of the patient's leg ulcer.

References:

Duchateau J, Delepesse G, Vrijen SR, Collet H. Beneficial effects of oral zinc supplementation on the immune response of old people. Am J Med 1981;70:1001-1004.

Morley JE. Nutritional status of the elderly. Am J Med 1986;81:679-695.

Sandstead HH, Henriksen LK, Greger JL, Prasad AS, Good RA. Zinc nutriture in the elderly in relation to taste acuity, immune response, and wound healing. Amer J Clin Nutr 1982;36:1046-1059.

Problem 18.

A 73-year-old woman is found to have squamous atypia on routine cervical Papanicolaou (pap) smear. Her last pap smear was done 40 years ago when she had her last child.

Questions:

1. What are the possible explanations for the cytologic findings?

2. What should be done?

Answers:

1.   Postmenopausal estrogen deficiency is associated with characteristic histologic changes in the cervix and vagina.   Thinning of mucosal squamous epithelium occurs, with decrease to complete loss of superficial cells, and predominance of intermediate or parabasal cells. The parabasal cells with large nuclei resemble the increased nuclear-to-cytoplasmic ratio seen in atypia. Atrophic cytology commonly includes inflammatory changes and the smear may be interpreted as showing squamous atypia.   Atypia implies dysplasia, which is a histologic precursor of carcinoma-in-situ.

Although the incidence of carcinoma-in-situ declines drastically after the age of 40, this is probably the result of mass screening programs, for the incidence of invasive cervical cancer increases somewhat with age. This patient has not been examined for 30 years and the possibility of true dysplasia is not ruled out.

2.   If no lesions are visible, some gynecologists recommend a short course of vaginal or oral estrogen, which will cause maturation of the epithelium and normalize the pap smear.   If atypia persists, further evaluation, including endometrial and cervical biopsy, should be done.

In actual practice, the incidence of false negatives is quite high, and is often due to improper smear collection or evaluation. This problem is, perhaps, more worrisome than the false-positive smear.

References:

Brown KH, Hammond CB.   Urogenital atrophy.   Obstet Gynecol Clin N Amer 1987;15:13-32.

Duguid HLD, Duncan ID, Currie J, Screening for cervical intraepithelial neoplasia in Dundee and Angus 1962-81 and its relation with invasive cervical cancer. Lancet 1985;2:1053-1056.

Hudson E, The prevention of cervical cancer: the place of the cytological smear test. Clin Obstet Gynaec 1985;12:33-51.

Weintraub NT, Violi E, Freedman ML.   Cervical cancer screening in women aged 65 and over.   J Amer Geriatr Soc 1987;35:870-875.

Problem 19.

A nonobese 79-year-old woman has a serum cholesterol level of 280 mg/dL. She says she follows a low-fat diet.

Questions:

1. What is the clinical significance of the cholesterol level?

2. Is drug therapy indicated?

Answer:

1. Cross-sectional studies reveal that serum cholesterol increases with age after age 20, reaching a plateau by midlife in men, and by age 70 in women, then declining slightly. The plateau and decline may represent a survival factor, in that fewer people with high cholesterol levels survive to late life. Although some longitudinal data confirm the decline, it is not known to what extent this represents dietary modifications that have taken place in recent years. High total cholesterol levels are not as important a risk factor for coronary artery disease in the elderly as they are in young and middle-aged adults, but the risk is still present. Determination of high (HDLC) or low-density lipoprotein cholesterol (LDLC) should be done. Levels of these subfractions correlate better with coronary risk in the elderly than do levels of total cholesterol, and their relative importance as predictors, compared to total cholesterol measurements, actually increases with age.

2. The correlation between serum cholesterol and coronary artery risk decreases strikingly with age, while the risk of myocardial infarction increases, so that factors other than serum cholesterol level are operating. Furthermore, studies demonstrating that lipid-lowering agents reduce the risk of coronary artery disease have included too few patients over 65 at baseline to draw conclusions about risk modification or the risk-benefit ratio of drug therapy in the elderly. Thus, decisions regarding drug treatment should be strictly individualized. If further laboratory evaluation of this patient reveals a plasma level of LDLC that is greater than 160 mg/dL, drug therapy should be considered, but only if blood levels are resistant to dietary therapy and exercise, and if the patient is highly motivated and functional. The agents of first choice are the anion exchange resins, cholestyramine and colestipol, which are not associated with important systemic side effects.

References:

Castelli WP, Garrison RJ, Wilson PWF, et al. Incidence of coronary artery disease and lipoprotein cholesterol levels: the Framingham study. JAMA 1986;256:2835-2838.

Gordon T, Castelli WP, Hjortland MC, Kannel WB, Dawber TR. High density lipoprotein as a protective factor against coronary heart disease: the Framingham Study. Am J Med 1979;62:707-714.

Hazzard WR. Disorders of lipoprotein metabolism. In: Andres R, Bierman EL, Hazzard WR, eds. Principles of geriatric medicine. New York: McGraw-Hill, 1985:764-775.

Hershcopf RJ, Elahi D, Andres R, et al. Longitudinal changes in serum cholesterol in man: an epidemiologic search for an etiology. J Chron Dis 1982;35:101-114.

Problem 20.

An 80-year-old Minnesota man had a Billroth II operation 20 years ago for a bleeding ulcer. He has had bilateral cataract excisions and wears aphakic spectacles, and also suffers from poor hearing. He has occasional heartburn and takes antacid (Mylanta) several times a day. Blood chemistries are normal except for slightly elevated alkaline phosphatase level. Complete blood count (CBC) is normal.

Questions:

1. He has an increased risk of fracture. Why?

2. What other blood tests are indicated?

3. What can be done?

4. What is meant by the term "osteopenia"?

Answers:

1. This patient has an increased risk of falling because he has perceptual deficits. Although he has had cataract surgery, his spectacles produce distortion and magnification, and leave him with suboptimal peripheral vision (see Case 27). His risk of fracture is due to the possibility that he has osteomalacia on top of age-related osteoporosis, the two conditions being radiographically indistinguishable when they co-occur. Gastric surgery is thought to impair vitamin D absorption. This man, furthermore, lives in a northern climate and may not receive adequate sunlight exposure to overcome this problem. The problem of osteomalacia in the elderly has been best studied in northern British Commonwealth countries where dairy products are not fortified with vitamin D, and where a seasonal variation in both vitamin D levels and hip fractures was first noted, but investigators feel that this problem occurs in American elderly as well, particularly those who are home-bound or institutionalized.

Blood tests are either normal or nonspecific in adult osteomalacia. In this patient the only clue is the slightly elevated alkaline phosphatase, an utterly nonspecific blood test in the elderly. Bone alkaline phosphatase reflects osteoblast function and is a measure of bone formation. Theoretically it should not be elevated in uncomplicated osteoporosis, which is associated with decreased osteoblast function. In osteomalacia, there is impaired mineralization of normal bone matrix, a process that can stimulate osteoblasts, even in senescent bone.

Mylanta and other phosphate-depleting, aluminum-containing antacids like Maalox and Riopan can theoretically increase the risk of osteomalacia in two ways--by depleting dietary phosphate and by increasing bone aluminum. Occasional use of these agents probably causes no clinical harm, but high-dose, longterm use should be discouraged.

2. A history of gastrectomy also increases the risk of vitamin B_{12} malabsorption, which may result in anemia and neurologic syndromes. Although the significance of a low serum B_{12} is the subject of controversy (see Problem 7), B_{12} level should be measured. Vitamin B_{12} deficiency can be present despite normal CBC. Vitamin D status should be determined by measuring serum 25-hydroxyvitamin D. This metabolite reflects dietary intake and sunlight production, and, because of its long serum half-life, indicates longterm status. Serum phosphate should be measured to rule out hypophosphatemia. Last, but hardly least, the physician should carefully investigate the reasons for his heavy ingestion of antacid.

3. Problems associated with determining B_{12} status have been discussed in Problem 7. If B_{12} status is equivocal, empiric treatment with B_{12} should be considered.

If vitamin D levels are normal, physiologic doses (400-800 IU per day or 50,000 IU once every 3 to 6 months) should be given to prevent osteomalacia. A limited course of higher doses is indicated if frank deficiency is demonstrated with a blood test.   Unrestricted use of his current antacid should be discouraged and might be replaced with monitored use of a calcium-containing antacid, after investigation of his "heartburn."

Sunlight exposure can normalize vitamin D status without producing hypervitaminosis.   During good weather, this patient should spend time outdoors; 15 to 30 minutes three times a week is probably all that is needed in light-skinned individuals.

4. "Osteopenia" is a general term that indicates decreased bone density. Osteopenia can be due to a number of disease processes, including osteoporosis, osteomalacia, myeloma, and other processes. Strictly speaking, it is more accurate to use the term "osteopenia" until clinical, biochemical, or occasionally, histologic criteria clarify what the disease process is.

References:

McKenna MJ, Freaney R, Meade A, Muldowney FP. Hypovitaminosis D and elevated serum alkaline phosphatase in elderly Irish people. Am J Clin Nutr 1985;41:101-109.

Nilsson BE, Westlin NE. The fracture incidence after gastrectomy. Acta Chir Scand 1971;137:533-534.

Omdahl JL, Garry PJ, Hunsaker LA, Hunt WC, Goodwin JS. Nutritional status in a healthy elderly population: Vitamin D. Am J Clin Nutr 1982;36:1225-1233.

Parfitt AM, Gallagher JC, Heaney RP, Johnston CC, Neer R, Whedon GD. Vitamin D and bone health in the elderly. Am J Clin Nutr 1982;36:1014-1031.

Weisman Y, Schen RJ, Eisenberg Z, et al. Single oral high-dose vitamin D_3 prophylaxis in the elderly. J Amer Geriat Soc 1986;34:515-518.

Problem 21.

An 83-year-old woman has abdominal pain after meals. There are no abdominal masses. Physical examination is normal. Abdominal ultrasound shows gallstones.

Question:

1. What is the diagnosis?

2. What should be done?

3. What if the gallstones had been discovered when spotted on a routine chest x-ray?

Answer:

1. The diagnosis is not necessarily gallbladder disease based on the demonstration of gallstones. Gallstones are present in 30 to 80% of people in their 80s at autopsy, the highest prevalence being in native Americans. Thus, gallstones are often silent and abdominal symptoms may be due to a number of other problems. Careful history, observation, and further tests should be done if presentation warrants.

2. If it is determined that the symptoms are due to gallstones, elective surgery should be considered. The risks of surgery increase with age, but the morbidity and mortality in emergency cholecystectomy are unacceptably high in the elderly.

3. "Silent" gallstones that are incidentally discovered in late life should stay where they are. Despite the claim that gallstones are associated with an increased risk of gallbladder cancer, this malignancy is not prevalent enough to warrant prophylactic cholecystectomy.

References:

Bateson MC, Bouchier IAD. Prevalence of gall stones in Dundee: a necropsy study. Brit Med J 1975;4:427-430.

Croker JR. Biliary tract disease in the elderly. Clin Gastroenterol 1985;14:773-809.

Gracie WA, Ransohoff DF. The natural history of silent gallstones: the innocent gallstone is not a myth. N Engl J Med 1982;307:798-800.

Hyams DE, Fox RA. The gastrointestinal system--the liver and biliary system. In: Brocklehurst JC, ed. Textbook of geriatric medicine and gerontology. Edinburgh: Churchill Livingstone, 1985:576-580.

Problem 22.

An elderly man has iron deficiency anemia. Barium enema shows extensive colonic diverticuli.

Question:

What is the cause of the iron deficiency?

Answer:

The iron deficiency has probably not been caused by diverticuli, unless he has a history of frank lower gastrointestinal bleeding. The incidence of diverticulosis increases with age, so that as many as 50% of 80-year-olds have diverticuli. Although massive bleeding can occur, diverticulosis is usually asymptomatic. Diverticular bleeding is arterial and when it occurs it is not occult. Thus, iron deficiency anemia or positive stool guaiac in the absence of significant overt bleeding should prompt a search for other gastrointestinal lesions. Stool guaiac may be positive, however, in symptomatic diverticulitis.

Another important cause of significant intestinal bleeding in the elderly is angiodysplasia (vascular ectasia) of the colon. The clinical presentation of this lesion ranges from intermittent guaiac positive stool to massive bleeding. Differentiation from diverticular bleeding may be difficult.

References:

Brandt LJ. Gastrointestinal disorders of the elderly. New York: Raven Press, 1984:281-324.

Gear JSS, Fursdon P, Nolan DJ, et al. Symptomless diverticular disease and intake of dietary fibre. Lancet 1979;1:511-514.

Parks TG. Post-mortem studies in the colon with special reference to diverticular disease. Proc Roy Soc Med 1968;62:932-934.

Problem 23.

A 69-year-old obese woman has a fasting triglyceride level of 422 mg/dL (N = 45-165). Serum cholesterol is 268 mg/dL. She is not diabetic, does not drink alcohol, and has no history of cardiac disease.

Questions:

1. What are the possible causes of the high triglyceride level?

2. What are the consequences?

3. What should be done?

Answers:

1. Although triglyceride levels increase with age, her triglyceride level is much higher than normal. The coexistence of a slightly elevated total cholesterol suggests familial hyperlipidemia, but secondary causes of hypertriglyceridemia need to be ruled out. Obesity and alcohol consumption may elevate triglyceride to this level. Thiazide diuretics and nonselective beta blockers also increase serum triglycerides, and may adversely affect cholesterol subfractions as well. These effects are thought to be mediated by counterregulatory phenomena such as increased production of insulin and catecholamines, which, in turn, act on hepatic lipid production. There is less information available regarding lipid profiles produced by other antihypertensive agents and loop diuretics. Hypertriglyceridemia can also be produced by exogenous estrogens, which decrease production of hepatic triglyceride lipase. Estrogen has a beneficial effect on cholesterol subfractions.

The fact that hypertriglyceridemia does not always occur in these settings implies that a genetic predisposition may need to be present.

2. It is not known whether lipid alterations by diuretics and antihypertensives have any clinical significance. Estrogens are thought by many to reduce the risk of arteriosclerotic disease in postmenopausal women, presumably by increasing high density lipoprotein (HDL) cholesterol.

The effect of hypertriglyceridemia per se has been the subject of great controversy. Although people with high triglyceride levels, including the elderly, have an increased risk of coronary artery disease, this risk may be due to associated risk factors, such as bad cholesterol profile, diabetes, and obesity. In the geriatric population, this increased coronary risk may be due to age alone. Triglyceride is not found in atheromas, and hypertriglyceridemia has not been demonstrated to enhance atherogenesis in animal studies or in carefully controlled human studies. On the other hand, multivariate analysis of certain epidemiologic studies indicates that presence of high triglycerides poses a distinct risk of coronary events in middle-aged subjects, unless HDL levels are very high. There is no theoretical explanation for this, although it has been suggested that other constituents of triglyceride-containing particles may be atherogenic or thrombogenic. An extremely high level of triglycerides (over 800 mg/dL), of course, increases the risk of acute pancreatitis.

3. The patient should be advised to exercise and lose weight, but the goal should be to lower low density lipoprotein (LDL) cholesterol, if it is found to be high, and to promote general health. If possible, lipid-altering drugs should be stopped. Drug therapy is not indicated for sole, moderate hypertriglyceridemia (250-500 mg/dL), even if it has not responded to diet and exercise. Marked elevations of triglyceride (roughly 800 mg/dL and above) increase the risk of pancreatitis and must be treated aggressively.

References:

Cambien F, Jacqueson A, Richard JL, Warnet JM, Ducimetiere P, Claude JR. Is the level of serum triglyceride a significant predictor of coronary death in "normocholesterolemic" subjects? Am J Epidemiol 1986;124:624-632.

Castelli WP. The triglyceride issue: a view from Framingham. Am Heart J 1986;112:432-437.

Consensus conference. Treatment of hypertriglyceridemia. JAMA 1984;251:1196-1200.

Hazzard WR. Biological basis of the sex differential in longevity. J Amer Geriatr Soc 1986;34:455-471.

Lardinois CK, Neuman SL. The effects of antihypertensive agents on serum lipids and lipoproteins. Arch Intern Med 1988;148:1280-1288.

Index